Making Bodies, Persons and Families

Edited by

Willemijn de Jong and Olga Tkach

Making Bodies, Persons and Families

Normalising Reproductive Technologies in Russia, Switzerland and Germany

Edited by

Willemijn de Jong and Olga Tkach

LIT

Cover picture: © Susi Kramer, Oberhof (CH), Cannes (F)

Proofreading: Sandy Ross (GB)
Layout: Christoph Schwager (CH)

Bibliographic information published by the Deutsche Nationalbibliothek
The Deutsche Nationalbibliothek lists this publication in the Deutsche Nationalbibliografie; detailed bibliographic data are available in the Internet at http://dnb.d-nb.de.

ISBN 978-3-643-80020-6

A catalogue record for this book is available from the British Library

Dufourstr. 31
CH-8008 Zürich
Tel. +41 (0) 44-251 75 05
Fax +41 (0) 44-251 75 06
e-Mail: zuerich@lit-verlag.ch
http://www.lit-verlag.ch

LIT VERLAG Dr. W. Hopf
Berlin 2009
Fresnostr. 2
D-48159 Münster
Tel. +49 (0) 2 51-620 32 22
Fax +49 (0) 2 51-922 60 99
e-Mail: lit@lit-verlag.de
http://www.lit-verlag.de

Distribution:
In Germany: LIT Verlag Fresnostr. 2, D-48159 Münster
Tel. +49 (0) 2 51-620 32 22, Fax +49 (0) 2 51-922 60 99, e-Mail: vertrieb@lit-verlag.de

In Austria: Medienlogistik Pichler-ÖBZ GmbH & Co KG
IZ-NÖ, Süd, Straße 1, Objekt 34, A-2355 Wiener Neudorf
Tel. +43 (0) 22 36-63 53 52 90, Fax +43 (0) 22 36-63 53 52 43, e-Mail: mlo@medien-logistik.at

In Switzerland: B + M Buch- und Medienvertriebs AG
Hochstr. 357, CH-8200 Schaffhausen
Tel. +41 (0) 52-643 54 30, Fax +41 (0) 52-643 54 35, e-Mail: order@buch-medien.ch

In the UK by: Global Book Marketing, 99B Wallis Rd, London, E9 5LN
Phone: +44 (0) 20 8533 5800 – Fax: +44 (0) 1600 775 663
http://www.centralbooks.co.uk/html

In North America by:

Transaction Publishers
New Brunswick (U.S.A.) and London (U.K.)

Transaction Publishers
Rutgers University
35 Berrue Circle
Piscataway, NJ 08854

Phone: +1 (732) 445 - 2280
Fax: + 1 (732) 445 - 3138
for orders (U. S. only):
toll free (888) 999 - 6778
e-mail: orders@transactionpub.com

Contents

Reproductive technologies, parenthood and families

Reproductive technologies, embryos and children

Medical scientific discourse and reproductive genetics

Appendix

Foreword: Making bodies, persons and families

The birth of Louise Brown in Oldham, near Manchester, in the northwest of England, in July of 1978, was the culmination of a lengthy process of investigation into the mechanisms of mammalian development and in particular the exploration of these processes in vitro. It was not until the postwar period that the ability to culture mammalian ova enabled reproductive biologists, embryologists, and medical scientists to observe and manipulate the very earliest stages of human life. These experiments were extremely labour-intensive and interdisciplinary. Nearly a decade separated the first successful fertilisation of human ova in vitro, at Cambridge in 1969, from the birth of the first offspring from this technique.

The field of reproductive biology is also notable, as Adele Clarke (1998) has noted in her pioneering account, *Disciplining Reproduction*, for both its proximity to social controversy and its wide variety of applications. The same techniques used to develop birth control led to the basic discoveries necessary for IVF. The ability to manipulate mammalian embryos in vitro was largely directed to agricultural applications for much of its contemporary history, and this area of applications in turn results from a shift in emphasis toward biological development that is one of the hallmarks of the modern life sciences.

Given the complex, and largely untold, history of clinical IVF, with its origins in agriculture and the veterinary sciences as much as in medicine and biology, we would expect it to have the strong regional character that social scientists have confirmed in the growing number of studies of assisted conception. The first studies of IVF in the late 1980s and early 1990s have been succeeded, like the delivery of IVF services, by a period of more rapid expansion in the late 1990s and early 'noughties', so that by the end of the first decade of the twenty-first century there is a comparatively well-established subdiscipline of what we might call biosocial studies of assisted reproduction.

Thus, along side the expansion of IVF as a predominantly private, increasingly international, and rapidly expanding sector of healthcare services are new studies, largely by social scientists, of IVF and other reproductive technologies in a wide range of settings – from fertility clinics in Egypt and Dubai (Inhorn), to IVF centres in Sri Lanka (Simpson), Israel (Kahn, Nahman), Turkey (Gurtin-Broadbent), India (Bharadwaj), Ecuador (Roberts), Canada (Burfoot), the United States (Thompson), and many other locations. These studies are important both for what they confirm about some of the general patterns of IVF provision, and for what they reveal about its specificity in different contexts. Hence, for example, the double-edged hope that IVF offers is a consistent theme in much research on IVF, confirming both the importance of IVF as a reproductive option, and the danger of its elusive promise of offspring, which, ultimately, fewer than half of those who attempt it will succeed in attaining. Similarly, while the global expansion of IVF services represents wider access to its potential rewards, the concomitant danger of new forms of reproductive stratification, such as those evident in the rise of 'reproductive tourism', point to the need to continue to document IVF provision and trace the increasing dispersions of reproductive 'products', namely valuable human gametes, and embryos.

It is all the more important to maintain a lively scholarly engagement with IVF due to its largely under-documented status as a medical practice. Despite the births of approximately five million offspring worldwide in the past thirty years – three quarters of whom will have been born in the past ten years, and half in the past five – IVF remains in many respects a very poorly understood phenomenon – socially, medically, demographically and biologically. As Debora Spar points out in her important book *The Baby Business*, the economies of IVF are chronically under-regulated, despite the enormous size of the IVF market. Hence, the task for social scientists is considerable.

Another key feature of the growing literature on IVF is the ability to begin to make important comparative distinctions within and between regions. Not only differences in the law, or religious attitudes toward IVF, but more subtle differences in concepts of parenthood, gender roles, and the values surrounding family formation can thus become apparent and more amenable to scrutiny.

It is for all of these reasons that the publication of the first anthology of scholarly research into new reproductive technologies in Switzerland and Russia is to be enthusiastically welcomed. This is the first volume to offer a sustained consideration by social scientists of Swiss and Russian assisted reproductive technologies, and the specific issues raised by assisted conception in these regions of the world. Bringing together twelve chapters of original scholarship by specialist researchers in this field represents an unprecedented accomplishment and will add immeasurably to the growing academic literature on this important field. As part of the wider project on new reproductive technologies in Eastern and middle Europe, and with particular implications for research on IVF in German speaking nations, this volume represents a timely contribution to a field that is destined to grow in importance.

Sarah Franklin
Professor of Social Studies of Biomedicine
BIOS Centre for the Study of Bioscience, Biomedicine and Society
London School of Economics

Introduction

Researching reproductive technologies in East and West

Willemijn de Jong and Olga Tkach

Technologies of assisted reproduction provide much food for thought and a plethora of lines of investigation – not the least from social and cultural researchers. This book sheds light on the hardly studied meanings of reproductive technologies and their normalisation related to constructions of the body, personhood, family, kinship and gender in Russia and Switzerland, and it provides further insights into these issues in Germany.

Procreation in the lab, without sexuality, has developed considerably since the birth of Louise Brown in Britain in 1978, and there has been a worldwide spread of in vitro fertilisation. Treatment options as well as related tests and research have become more and more diversified because of scientific progress. As these procedures touch upon extremely emotional and morally contentious issues of life itself, including death, they polarise public and personal opinions. Thus it is not surprising that these issues have been hotly debated in the media, and remain a burning issue.

Switzerland is a country with strict legal rules regarding assisted reproduction, as is Germany. Almost every week some article on this issue features in Swiss daily and weekly newspapers and magazines, and related films have been broadcasted on German-speaking television channels occasionally in the last couple of years. This public debate is often grounded in legislative policy that has to be decided through creating public awareness of medical treatments. Paradoxically, public social acceptance of reproductive technologies is increasing, but at the same time its use is imbued with secrecy and taboos, at least in Switzerland. Those under treatment often deal with these matters only in their most intimate relationships. In Russia, a country with little legal regulation of reproductive technologies, the media debate on assisted reproduction is tinged with collective fears, misunderstandings and moralistic statements derived from the newness of the phenomenon. But issues such as the governmental programs aimed at raising the birthrate in Russia by these technologies are positively valued. This book tries to fathom the social and cultural background of the anxieties and hopes related to these technologies.

How can we define assisted reproductive technologies? This term is commonly considered synonymous with new reproductive technologies (NRTs), but in recent years the former has become more prevalent, conveniently abbreviated as ARTs (Strathern 2005; Thompson 2005; Inhorn and Birenbaum-Carmeli 2008). In a narrow sense, these technologies comprise procedures of fertilisation outside the human body: in vitro fertilisation (IVF) with patients' own gametes, which may include intracytoplasmic sperm injection (ICSI), or with sperm, egg and embryo donation by third parties, and surrogacy. In everyday understandings, these procedures as well as artificial insemination by husband (AIH) or by donor (AID) are often called artificial fertilisation. In a broader social scientific sense, ARTs also encompass prenatal testing, including pre-implantation genetic diagnostics (PGD), birthing techniques such as Caesarian section, as well as preventive technologies of contraceptives and abortion (Saetnan et al. 2000). Assisted reproductive technologies are also strongly related to the medical and biological fields of stem cell research, genetic research and cloning (Franklin and Lock 2003). However, in this volume we refer to ARTs in the former, narrower sense, unless indicated otherwise. Although many of these contributions are concerned with the use of ARTs related to bodily infertility, it should be stressed that they are also more and more used to build families in cases in which there is no medical diagnosis of infertility (Thompson 2005).

Shared Interests, divided contexts

In Anglophone countries, social and cultural studies of ARTs and related subjects have mushroomed since the 1990s. The first ethnographies published have focused on Britain and the United States, but soon expanded to ARTs in specific national and local contexts, all around the world and across many religious backgrounds. In the meantime research on ARTs have proliferated especially in the fields of social studies on science and technology, studies of the body and gender, medical anthropology, and new kinship studies (cf. e.g. Franklin 1995; Sharp 2000; Inhorn and Birenbaum-Carmeli 2008).

The research on which this volume is based was particularly inspired by studies in Britain and the United States which show that ARTs have destabilising social effects with which individuals and societies have to cope. Notions and practices regarding kinship and family, particularly subjectivities of motherhood and fatherhood, personhood of embryos, and the body and its gendered specificity are restabilised in different ways. In general, in Eastern Europe the social and cultural meanings and effects of ARTs are heavily understudied compared to other countries in the industrialised world (but see Hofman 2005). The same applies to Switzerland (but see Gross and Honer 1990; Arni 2008). In Germany, research on this subject started in the mid-1990s but with respect to Russia and Switzerland, this book represents a pioneering exploration.

The contributions are the results of a joint research project entitled 'New Reproductive Technologies and the Making of Bodies, Persons and Families in Russia and Switzerland'. It took place from January 2006 until December 2008 within the program of Scientific Cooperation between Eastern Europe and Switzerland (SCOPES 2005-2008) and was funded by the Swiss National Science Foundation (SNSF) and the Swiss Development Cooperation (SDC) of the Federal Department for Foreign Affairs. The participating scholars from the Russian team were Olga Brednikova, who led the team, Nadya Nartova and Olga Tkach, who are research fellows at the Centre for Independent Social Research in St. Petersburg. Participants in the Swiss team were Willemijn de Jong, who was the head of the project, Shahanah Schmid, Andrea Früh and Zora Schaad. During the project they were all affiliated with the Department of Social and Cultural Anthropology at the University of Zurich.

Our research project had the following objectives. The first of these was to investigate the processes of development and distribution of ARTs in Russia and Switzerland. Main goals were to examine the production, representations, and functions of the gendered body, the person and the family in the discourses and social practices related to ARTs. This project has further attempted to probe the boundaries of moral categories and judgements about ARTs in order to examine discursive strategies that justify the use of ARTs. As a first research question we asked: How have ARTs in Russia and Switzerland influenced the meanings and practices related to the body, the person, and the family, and what are the social implications? This is also a crucial question in the other contributions to this volume.

Despite our shared interests, our approach – studying ARTs in two very different contexts – was not easy. The disparities between the two countries are enormous, not the least being the sheer size difference, but the gulf in socio-economic welfare and the totally different social history must also be considered, among other differences. Given that even superficially similar countries such as the Scandinavian states developed widely different legal and discursive approaches to ARTs (Norden 2006), it is no wonder that there are many differences in the ways these technologies became a social phenomenon in Russia and Switzerland.

It was clear from the onset that a conventional cross-national and cross-cultural comparison between these countries would lead to unsatisfactory results, as we would grasp the investigated phenomena only superficially. Therefore, we decided to work with the analytic concept of normalisation. Regarding our theoretical perspective, all of us refer to theories of practice in one way or another. For example, the processes of normalisation and legitimation are particularly visible in the realm of ARTs because of a lack of preexisting, unreflected doxa, in the sense of Bourdieu, which thus necessitates explicit deliberation in order to establish orthodoxies and heterodoxies. Furthermore, referring to Foucault, we are aware that strategies of normalisation are particularly relevant in disciplinary relationships and institutions.

Although we did not follow a classically comparative approach, conducting our research in two different cultural settings in parallel still proved to be productive. It became easier to discover relevant issues and to improve the rigour of our individual research than if we had conducted a project in a mono-cultural context. We started from the presumption that the normalisation of ARTs is a major social and cultural mechanism in that ARTs and their social effects are incorporated into existing ideas and practices and at the same time, the existing social order is transformed in the course of this process. As a second research question we therefore asked: What kind of discursive and practical techniques or strategies of normalisation can be found in the context of ARTs, and how are they legitimised?

Methodologically, we conducted qualitative research. We used textual material, in particular newspaper and scientific articles, as well as religious documents, and material from interviews with mothers and fathers of children born thanks to ARTs and with persons without direct experiences with these treatments. Some of us relied on additional material of participant observation in selected families with ART children. As we could conduct only a small-scale research project because of budget restrictions, we decided to focus, as a first step, more strongly on cultural meanings in discourses and individual views than on the social practices of actors, which would have required more ethnographic interviews and observation. This is also the reason why the contributions of the Russian scholars deal with the discourse on ARTs in the print media.

Both teams strongly benefited from the cooperation in the research project. It enabled us to conduct innovative comparative research and to conduct exchange visits to get to know other scholars and scientific institutes. The annual workshops we organised, two in St. Petersburg and two in Zurich, were excellent opportunities to set up a common research framework and to discuss differences and similarities of both situations as well as the research results. Further participants in the workshops were Michi Knecht and Bettina Bock von Wülfingen, scholars from the Humboldt University in Berlin with comprehensive experience in social studies on ARTs in Germany (Knecht 2007, Bock von Wülfingen 2007). Moreover, we benefited from scientific exchanges with Sarah Franklin from the BIOS Centre at the London School of Economics and Political Science (LSE), a leading researcher in the field of social studies of ARTs and genetics in Britain (Franklin 1997, 2007). The latter two scholars also contributed to this book. Thus, this volume gives an account of joint social research on ARTs in Russia, Switzerland, and Germany as well.

What is the relevance of these kinds of studies and of scientific cooperation between Eastern and Central European countries, or between East and West? The research of the Russian scholars is a pioneer project in the field of social studies on ARTs in Russia. The academic papers and seminars resulting from this research initiated an academic debate on these issues, which is important and urgent for the current situation in Russia. Research findings were also exchanged through seminars with activists and practitioners. The Russian research team members hope this collaboration will assist them not only in solving certain social problems related to the spread of reproductive technologies, but also to redefine the predominantly negative attitude to the newness of ARTs in Russian society. Both teams tried to contribute to the intellectual debate on social issues of ARTs in an academic context, and several project participants also have begun to disseminate their research results to the general public.

Normalising ARTs, bodies, persons and families

The volume consists of four thematic sections about ARTs and their normalisation: the body and gender; parenthood and families; person-like embryos and children; and the medicalised discourse of reproductive medicine and genetics. Before that, in a further introductory chapter the conceptual frame of the contributions is discussed and in a first section the national contexts of the research are sketched.

In the next introductory chapter, Willemijn de Jong discusses the analytical concept of normalisation referring to Charis Thompson's (2005) important monograph on ARTs in the United States entitled

Making Parents: The Ontological Choreography of Reproductive Technologies. An expansion and differentiation is proposed, and more reflections on power, the relationship of science and religion and what remains abnormal are advocated. All the authors take Thompson's concept of normalisation as a starting point, and apply this concept more or less critically in their contributions, or distance themselves from it and look at normalisation in other ways, depending on their theoretical viewpoint and the logic of their data.

In the section on national regimes of reproductive technologies, Olga Brednikova, Nadya Nartova and Olga Tkach present a contemporary background of ARTs in Russia. This chapter outlines the development of IVF and other forms of assisted reproduction and their institutional infrastructure. It also discusses the problematisation of ARTs in the public, not exclusively scientific and medical, realm. The overview describes how, and in what forms, reproductive technologies found their way into the legislature.

Shahanah Schmid provides an overview of the regulation of ARTs in Switzerland from the early 1980s onwards, and illustrates the legal situation at present. It can best be described as socially restrictive whilst technologically relatively permissive. The overview includes information on the frequencies of treatments, which have roughly doubled per decade, and their success rates. The current situation in Germany regarding regulation and treatment frequencies is also briefly discussed. These chapters, as well as a table in the appendix, show that the conditions of ARTs especially in Russia on the one hand, and Switzerland and Germany on the other, are quite different indeed.

The first chapter in the section on bodies, gender and ARTs by Nadya Nartova concerns body production and normalisation in ART discourse in Russian print media. The focus is on the most problematic practices within Russian media debate: on surrogate motherhood and sperm donorship. The process of impregnation becomes autonomous, and the reproductive body becomes a service provider. Female and male bodies are constituted and normalised within this context in opposite ways. This leads to the formation of opposite types of subjects in the sphere of ARTs.

In the second chapter of this section, Andrea Früh distinguishes four distinct categories of normalisation strategies applied by women before, during or after their IVF treatments: reproduction of the nuclear family; naturalisation; normalisation within the clinical setting; and gendered normalisation. These strategies are used by individual women and in an individual way; but implicitly or explicitly they refer to collective, societal norms and are always embedded in public discourses.

The third section deals with parenthood, families and ARTs. Zora Schaad shows that reproductive technologies in Switzerland hold the potential to fulfil the 'natural' wish for a child but often count as 'artificial'. Normalisation processes entail dealing with one's social surroundings and are influenced by norms that exist around procreation. Normalisation is varied within the child searching process. An orientation towards the 'normal biography', strategies of (non-)disclosure, and efforts of embedding the situation are identified.

In the second chapter of this section, Olga Tkach distinguishes the concepts of kinship, parenthood and family, derived from the application of ARTs and represented in Russian print media. Analysis is focused on the most prominent variants of donorship programs illustrated with argumentations and stories about the tricky process of defining kinship. The author traces, how temporarily fragmented fatherhood and motherhood as constructed in public discourse of ARTs are finally integrated into general social parenthood.

The third section of the volume is dedicated to embryos and emerging children in the context of ARTs. Willemijn de Jong deals with embryo meanings of Swiss medical and religious experts and mothers, as well as practices used to normalise the newness of ARTs and relatedness with the embryo. It is shown that normalisations based on the biological, the natural, the social and the sacred retraditionalise existing kinship and gender orders, but also enable or promote innovation. Depending upon individuals' scientific and religious beliefs and their own biographic experience, embryos can become surprisingly full persons and relatives, or incipient ones.

Olga Brednikova focuses in her chapter on subjectivity and the production of 'otherness' of ART children in Russian print media. These 'ersatz' and cyborg children have an ambivalent status and a contradictory subjectivity: their otherness is stressed, at the same time they are normalised and it is their 'mission' to reconstruct the broken social order and to become a member in the genetic chain of succession. An emergent market discourse holds potential for transformation and redefinition of social norms related to ARTs.

The last section deals with medicalised discourse and ARTs. Shahanah Schmid explores science as culture, using medical scientific publications as material. Quantification is shown to be an important way in which scientific culture deals with new problems. The article also discusses what it means when fertility treatment, as well as fertility, is set as standard. It is pointed out that reference to nature need not always mean the same, and that it is necessary to explore culturally which function naturalisation – in relation to normalisation – has in diverse contexts and settings.

The chapter by Bettina Bock von Wülfingen evaluates international experts' discourses promoting new reproductive and genetic technologies in German print media from 1995 until 2003 and their fitting with the German context. Normalisation in this study refers to the notion of bridgeheads and concerns. The notion of the bridgehead is a term for concepts which link the unknown 'new' technology to well-known (here: accustomed) phenomena in the specific cultural context. Additionally, new technology meets concerns which their promoters address in the introduction of technology.

Acknowledgements

We thank the SNSF and the SDC for their financial support of our research, including the publication of this volume. Furthermore, we are grateful for infrastructure and support from the Department of Social and Cultural Anthropology at the University of Zurich and the Centre for Independent Social Research in St. Petersburg. We also thank all the people who helped us with collecting the empirical data, particularly informants who shared their often delicate experiences with us. Michi Knecht and Bettina Bock von Wülfingen contributed to the research process with fruitful ideas, theoretical and methodological, and they gave insightful comments on our presentations and papers, which we strongly appreciate. We kindly thank Sarah Franklin for her references and for her contribution to this book. Her work was a rich source of inspiration for our project. Furthermore, we are grateful for the careful proof reading by Sandy Ross and for the skilful work on the layout by Christoph Schwager which makes the reading of our book hopefully also a pleasant endeavour.

References

Arni, C. (2008) Menschen machen aus Akt und Substanz: Prokreation und Vaterschaft im reproduktionsmedizinischen und literarischen Experiment, *Gesnerus. Swiss Journal of the History of Medicine and Science* 65: 196-224.

Bock von Wülfingen, B. (2007) *Genetisierung der Zeugung: Eine Diskurs- und Metaphernanalyse reproduktionsgenetischer Zeugung.* Bielefeld: transcript Verlag.

Franklin, S. (1997) *Embodied Progress: A Cultural Account of Assisted Conception.* London, New York: Routledge.

Franklin, S. (1995) Science as culture, cultures of science, *Annual Review of Anthropology*, 24: 163-184.

Franklin, S. (2007) *Dolly Mixtures: The Remaking of Genealogy.* Durham: Duke University Press.

Franklin, S. and Lock, M (2003) Animation and cessation: the remaking of life and death in S. Franklin and M. Lock (eds) *Remaking Life and Death: Toward an Anthropology of the Biosciences*. Philadelphia: University of Philadelphia Press: 3-22.

Gross, P. and Honer, A. (1990) Multiple Elternschaften: Neue Reproduktionstechnologien, Individualisierungsprozesse und die Veränderung von Familienkonstellationen, *Soziale Welt* 41(1): 97-116.

Hofmann, H. (Hg.) (2005) *Biopolitik grenzenlos. Stimmen aus Polen*. Herbolzheim: Centaurus Verlag.

Inhorn, M.C. and Birenbaum-Carmeli, D. (2008) Assisted reproductive technologies and culture change, *Annual Review of Anthropology*, 37: 177-196.

Knecht, M. (2007) Spätmoderne Genealogien: Praxen und Konzepte verwandtschaftlicher Bindung und Abstammung, in S. Beck, N. Çil, S. Hess, M. Kloth, und M. Knecht (Hg.) *Verwandtschaft machen: Reproduktionsmedizin und Adoption in Deutschland und der Türkei.*

Saetnan, A.R., N. Oudshoorn and M. Kirejczyk (eds.) (2000) *Bodies of Technology: Women's Involvement with Reproductive Medicine*. Columbus, Ohio: Ohio State University.

Norden (Nordic Committee on Bioethics) (2006) *Assisted Reproduction in Nordic Countries. A Comparative Study of Policies and Regulation*. Copenhagen: Nordic Council.

Sharp, L.A. (2000) The commodification of the body and its parts, *Annual Review of Anthropology*, 29: 287-328.

Strathern, M. (2005) *Kinship, Law and the Unexpected: Relatives Are Always a Surprise*. Cambridge: Cambridge University Press.

Thompson, C. (2005) *Making Parents: The Ontological Choreography of Reproductive Technologies*. London, Cambridge, MA: MIT Press.

Reproductive technologies and the concept of normalisation

Willemijn de Jong

> I think that normalization, that disciplinary normalizations, are increasingly in conflict with the juridical system of sovereignty; the incompatibility of the two is increasingly apparent; there is a greater and greater need for a sort of arbitrating discourse, for a sort of power and knowledge that has been rendered neutral because its scientificity has become sacred. And it is precisely in the expansion of medicine that we are seeing – I wouldn't call it a combination of, a reduction of – but a perpetual exchange or confrontation between the mechanics of discipline and the principle of right. The development of medicine, the general medicalization of behavior, modes of conduct, discourses, desires, and so on, is taking place on the front where the heterogeneous layers of discipline and sovereignty meet.
> Michel Foucault, *Society Must Be Defended*, 2003: 39

> (...) the modernities reflected in ART are both sacralised and scientific, actual and imaginary, promissory and disappointing. In sum, here [in 'the West'], as elsewhere, IVF reveals their hybridity and their importance to an anthropology of what is biological, as well as what is spiritual, modern, technological, or scientific.
> Sarah Franklin, *Origin stories revisited: IVF as an anthropological project*, 2006: 553

Although increasingly publicly debated, assisted reproductive technologies (ARTs) such as in vitro fertilisation (IVF) and intracytoplasmic sperm injection (ICSI) are medical treatments that are still imbued by taboos and by the silencing of the issue of unwanted childlessness by the people concerned. Though reproduction in the lab is not considered abnormal anymore, it is still fraught with ambivalence. This is not only the case in countries like India or Egypt (Bharadwaj 2003, Inhorn 2002), but also in the West, as the contributions in this volume show. One of the themes of this collection is how different actors cope with the ways that ARTs, and related technologies and research, displace ideas and practices of the body, personhood, kinship and the family through its cultural and social effects. In other words, we are concerned with how the newness of reproductive technologies is normalised. To analyse these issues we turn to 'reflexive comparison' as I propose to call it; that is, comparison with the help of a critically reflected joint focus and concept, namely normalisation. In the articles in this volume we try to give answers to the following questions: What kind of discursive and practical techniques or strategies of normalisation can be found in the context of reproductive technologies, and how are they legitimised?

In social practice, the innovative social and cultural potential of ARTs is not at all exhausted, in many cases a range of as yet unexplored possibilities remain – this is a prominent theme in research literature (Franklin 1997; Thompson 2005). Several contributions in this volume show that efforts of normalisation actually reify existing, earlier conditions of bodies, gender and the family. Other contributions indicate that in public discourse, and in individual thinking and action, ARTs are used to redefine intimate social relationships and the relationships to bodies and the selves, generating new subjectivities. The aim of this chapter is not to go deeper into these questions, but to discuss the concept of normalisation and its performative repertoires, as developed in recent literature. This chapter also examines the kinds of shifts in meaning and practices of basic elements of the social order that ARTs effect, especially the kin relationship of motherhood and fatherhood. The anthropological perspective of this introductory article overlaps with the analytical concepts and strategies of other contributions in this anthology, but in some of them alternative concepts are used.

Normalisation as the normal and the normative

Charis Thompson's studies are a good point of departure to look at normalisation. She is one of the leading scholars in the field of social studies on ARTs. In her book *Making Parents: The Ontological Cho-*

reography of Reproductive Technologies (2005), as well as in previous articles, Thompson (formerly Cussins, 1998), examines techniques of normalisation in an infertility clinic in the United States. Her ethnographic study shows that during the processes of IVF, including ICSI, patients apply different strategies to normalise the destabilisation of motherhood or fatherhood, and gender identities, caused by ARTs. Generally, Thompson's reflections are based on Foucault, Goffman, science studies and feminist studies. Concerning ARTs, she continues the pioneering anthropological work done in this field by Marilyn Strathern, Sarah Franklin and others in Britain (e.g. Strathern [1993] 1999, 1995; Franklin 1997). In this chapter I will examine Thompson's concept of normalisation, and based on theoretical reflections and my empirical study in this volume I will propose some revisions.

Thompson (2005: 80) defines the social process of normalisation thus:

> Normalization includes the means by which 'new data' (new patients, new scientific knowledge, new staff members, new instruments, new administrative constraints) are incorporated into pre-existing procedures and objects of the clinic. It also includes the ways in which the grid of what is already there is produced, recognized, reproduced, and changed over time. This use of the concept of normalization incorporates both 'normal' and 'normative' (...).

It is interesting that normalisation is conceptualised as a two-way process: new phenomena are absorbed into the existing order, and the existing order – most obviously with respect to issues regarding kinship and gender – is also changed through these new phenomena. What is missing, however, are theoretical reflections on new data that are either temporarily absorbed or not incorporated at all into the existing structures of the clinic, and into the existing social and cultural structures beyond the clinic – phenomena that remain abnormal and against the norms for the time being (de Jong 2008). Empirically, normalisation is examined in the context of the clinic, specifically how women's body parts come to represent the couple during the treatment and the way treatment cycles tend to be repeated through the clinic's statistical culture. Moreover, presentations of self and couplehood are dealt with, including the repair of threatened identity, and complicity with the epistemic and 'technical things' of the treatment.

Thompson argues that normalisation in the clinic 'grows from versions of life, parenthood, and fertility that are already present in the wider culture'. She (2005: 115) suggests that 'social categories and techniques develop together and thereby change what life, parenting, and fertility mean in cultures with infertility clinics'. Although in the contributions in this volume we mainly look at normalisation in contexts other than infertility clinics – e.g. in public contexts of media and science discourse and in personal contexts of domestic relationships in which meanings and practices regarding ARTs, kinship and gender are created and negotiated – Thompson's study is useful as a main point of departure for our common conceptual frame. The production of normalisation is open to diverse theoretical groundings and methodological approaches, and seems to be applicable to the Russian, the Swiss and the German context.

'Statistification' and routinisation as normalising practices

Statistics are an important means of normalising, or making things seem the same. Thompson (2005: 109, emphasis added) even argues that 'without the statistical justificatory system working, all the other *repertoires of normalization* and *making things relevantly the same* cannot be calibrated and validated'. Our contributions show that this is not only the case in the clinic, but also in public discourse and in everyday life.

Referring to Karin Knorr-Cetina, Thompson (2005: 104) demonstrates that the entire epistemic culture of infertility clinics is based on the production of statistics. The success of a reproductive procedure is expressed not so much as a matter of experience, than as a statistical probability. This statistically based epistemic culture, in conjunction with the lack of alternative operationalisations, leads to what she (2005:94) calls a 'culture of perseverance in clinics'. As a rule, patients are hardly able to stop the treatments by themselves, as Thompson found. Franklin (1997) has documented the same phenomenon in Britain. Any statistical numbers achieved from diagnostic tests or surgery can infinitely nurture hopes of a future with a (further) child:

> The combination of cumulative probabilities plus fine-tuning means that the treatment plan is infinite. Cycles can always be ruled crucially not the same and so not counted; statistics will always say that this might be the time that the same procedure will work. (Thompson 2005: 95)

For convenience, I suggest calling this practice of normalisation 'statistification'. New patients are judged based on 'statistics as a normative epistemology' (Thompson, 2005: 104). At the same time, the treatment cycles of patients, not the patients as individuals, contribute to further statistification – and thus normalisation – of childlessness and reproductive medicine. Thompson (2005: 106) also gives evidence that the compilation of statistics, which are handwritten, is a problematic endeavour. 'At weekly team meetings the parameters of statistics become negotiable', and she concludes 'statistics are generated, recorded, and manipulated in several places, and a fairly large proportion of the lab technician's time is spent on them'.

A further practice of normalisation is routinisation. This practice particularly applies to the medical personnel in context of the clinic and reproductive medicine. According to Thompson, normalisation includes routinisation, primarily in terms of skilled local knowledge exercised by medical personnel and patients in conjunction with medical technologies. Medical personnel possess routinised skills that implicate the enactment of epistemic norms of seeing, feeling, and knowing, according to a certain division of labour, e.g. reading ultrasound scans or carrying out pelvic exams or surgery. In this sense, the clinic displays a 'culture of skills' (Thompson, 2005: 102). For example, when reading a scan screen, follicle counts are used to decide what is natural, and to make a diagnosis about what is normal or abnormal. Routinisation is also used in connection with administrative matters, which she (2005: 80) calls 'bureaucratic routinisation', and also includes efficient handling of different time-scales: bureaucratic, cyclical and biological.

Naturalisation and socialisation as normalising practices

Normalisation not only encompasses statistification and routinisation, it also includes naturalisation according to Thompson's theoretical frame: 'naturalization (...) is an important part of normalization' and 'what is normal is often stabilized by what is natural in this site [infertility clinic]' (2005: 80, 81). As an example, she mentions that the clinic accepts that patients present themselves as stable heterosexual couples because a 'mother-and-father family' is normative for the clinic. These statements already suggest her (2005: 81) two-fold definition of normalisation: 1) 'the rendering of states of affairs and facts in a scientific or biological idiom' and 2) 'the means by which aspects of the site are rendered unproblematic or self-evident'. The fusion of two very different components of meaning in the concept of normalisation seems rather problematic to me, especially if we want to use naturalisation as an analytic concept. Whereas the first strategy is specific and focused only on scientific metaphors which seem to be equated with biological metaphors, the second can include a whole range of different idioms, based on many different kinds of reasoning. I will return to this problematic stance later.

Thompson (2005: 82) also refers to naturalisation as socionaturalisation, to underline that this is a social practice. For example, as an ethnographer, Thompson herself had to undergo socionaturalisation in the clinic, which was brought about by wearing a white coat like a medical doctor, among other things. Normalising practices of 'making self-evident' not only create the acceptable ethnographer in the clinical setting, but first and foremost they create the 'good patient', i.e. a white, middle- or upper-income patient couple.

Disciplinary norms of heterosexuality, ability to pay, appropriate comportment and compliance are enforced in the clinic in specific ways. This specificity is at the same time a source of change:

> This translation of societal norms into the everyday practice of the clinic in turn reinforced and changed (through applying them in new contexts) the various expressions of these norms in wider society. (Thompson 2005: 85)

There has been a shift in the conceptualisation of the 'good patient'. At the end of the 1990s, there was decreasing emphasis in patient selection upon 'high incomes, homes they would provide future children' (Thompson 2005: 89), and more concern for patients' rights, needs, or the right timing for reproduction. Thompson documents this subtle shift from children's rights to adults' reproductive rights, which was accompanied by a change of ethical frame: from social interventionism to privacy. In contrast to adoption and surrogacy, IVF is increasingly treated as a matter of reproductive privacy. I suppose that this may also be a reason why it is not easy to free ARTs from their taboo character. In fact, this new way of thinking about ARTs may even reinforce such reactions. In this context of decreasing explicit socioeconomic norms, Thompson (2005: 90-91) observes an increase in the use of biological norms. For instance, not only women's menstrual cycle is examined to diagnose infertility today and to decide about a treatment, but also many other bodily phenomena are tested, such as ovarian response after the use of drugs to produce eggs for IVF.

Assisted reproductive technologies lead to the destabilisation of bodily, kinship and gender identities, as Thompson's study shows, but they also assist in the repair or restabilisation of these identities by the subjects themselves and by practitioners in the social context of the clinic. With respect to the restabilisation of gender identity in the course of procreative treatments, Thompson (2005: 145-178) detects not only 'naturalizing strategies' but also 'denaturalizing' or 'socializing strategies' in cases of egg donation and gestational surrogacy that involve kin and friends as third parties. At issue is the disambiguation of kinship and making clear who the real mother (or father) is, and repairing male (and female) identity.

In her investigations of making kinship, particularly motherhood, in the clinic, Thompson (2005: 171) shows that persons who are involved in the process of procreative intent as a third party, by providing eggs or use of the uterus for gestation, are mostly dekinned,[1] whereas the relationship between the intended mother and the future child is kinned. We should add that a kind of dekinning may also take place in the relationship with practitioners (Strathern 2001).

> The alignment of procreative intent and biological kinship is achieved over time through a mixed bag of everyday and more formal strategies for naturalizing and socializing particular traits, substances, precedents, and behaviours. (Thompson 2001: 145)

Regarding naturalising strategies, Thompson finds that the people concerned primarily stress criteria of biogenetic substance and biologised notions of descent. This finding is supported by previous studies of American kinship (Schneider 1968). But in certain contexts, other aspects come to the fore, and this basic biogenetic understanding becomes denaturalised or socialised. Socialising practices are particularly obvious regarding gestation in the United States. Gestation is increasingly socialised and de-privatised in that it is equated with the care of the child after its birth. This is advanced by fetal monitoring, enabled by visualising techniques such as sonography, and by a general child-based perspective of human reproduction.

In the case of gestational surrogacy, socialising strategies are also often at work, but only related to gestation, not to fertilisation. Thus, we have to take into account that the phases of gestation and fertilisation can be differently normalised regarding the relatedness of mother and child. With egg donation, it is just the opposite: gestation is renaturalised in that the biological nature of kinship is emphasised. Even though there is no genetic link, fertilisation is socialised. Giovanna, an Italian American woman, chose the eggs of a friend from the same ethnic group, arguing that they are emotionally close, both have Italian mothers and are from the same background socially and culturally. This would provide 'enough genetic similarity', she said (Thompson 2005: 156). Ethnicity is understood here as a national and natural category of Italian Americanness, transported by genes. This woman socialises the culturally important idea that the same genes are important for descent, particularly for a parent-child relationship. With regard to this example of 'socializing genetics', Thompson (2005: 157) also reflects on the overlapping of nature and culture:

> Genes figure in Giovanna's kinships reckoning because there is a chain of transactions between the natural and cultural that not only grounds the cultural in the natural but gives the natural its explanatory power by its links to culturally relevant categories.

Thompson observed several cases in which genetics were 'coded back' to socioeconomic factors and thus a deessentialising of genetics took place. In this context she formulates one of her main propositions regarding Euro-American kinship and ARTs:

> Eliding ethnonational and race- and class-based categories with natural grounds for designating kinship is a strategy fundamental to bilateral, blood-based kinship systems. (Thompson 2005: 172)

Based on theses findings, she concludes that in modern medicine practioners and patients 'flexibly manage the choreography between the natural and the cultural' (2005: 177). She goes on to suggest that

> sometimes important political and ontological work is done by denaturalizing what has previously been taken to be natural and deterministic; sometimes the reverse is necessary.

Supernaturalisation or sacralisation as a further normalising strategy

In exploring the choreography and innovativeness of processes of naturalisation, Thompson has been inspired by *Naturalizing Power*, a volume editied by Sylvia Yanagisako and Carol Delaney (1995). These authors (1995:1) define naturalizing power as 'ways in which differentials of power come already embedded in culture', based on the assumption that 'power appears natural, inevitable, even god-given'. At issue is the 'naturalisation of identities and social bonds by claiming for them an autonomy from human social agency' based on nature, biology, or god as a supernatural force. These are the non-human phenomena that legitimise 'hierarchies of difference in which power relations are embedded' (Yanagisako and Delaney, 1995: 20). The authors themselves focus in particular on our own origin myths: the religious account of Genesis and secular scientific accounts of evolutionary theory. They advocate that we explore how both kinds of origin stories have naturalised our world view, and argue that secular evolutionary accounts still entail aspects of the supernatural or the 'god-given quality' when they naturalise the orders of creation.[2] Implicated in this approach is the construction of power as a self-evident phenomenon in the fields of gender, family, sexuality, race, nation and religion. The second criteria of Thompson's definition mentioned above, that is, ways of making self-evident, is here at issue. Whereas Yanagisako and Delaney include naturalisation through a supernatural idiom, it is striking – and it seems restricting – that Thompson only focuses on a scientific or biological idiom.

Thompson's focus is on knowledge practices that normalise the natural – biological kinship and gender – which gets more or less re-naturalised or socialised according to the bodily and social context. This is quite another point of departure than a focus on knowledge practices about normalising power conditions, especially kin and gender relationships, which become naturalised or supernaturalised. Looked at through this lens, it is striking that power is hardly an issue in Thompson's study. And how about supernaturalising or sacralisation, as I call a strategy or practice based on a spiritual or religious idiom?

Thompson deals with the sacred embryo in the last chapter of her book. Yet, surprisingly, religious rhetorical strategies and other practices of the actors involved in ARTs do not seem to be of relevance, theoretically and empirically, with respect to normalisation. I only found one passage in the book that can give a theoretical clue to how Thompson conceptualises the relationship of normalisation and supernaturalising strategies, besides naturalising and socialising. Regarding the 'epistemic culture based on statistics' which leads to a 'culture of perseverance' (2005: 94), Thompson talks about the general lack of alternative operationalisations. In this context she mentions that she met only one woman in the clinic who gave up treatment by herself, without external pressure, which she explains thus:

> The unusual commodity that this woman appeared to possess was a network for interpreting her infertility outside of the medical one. She credited her Mormon religion. At this point in her treatment, it was as powerful as the medical operationalization. (Thompson 2005: 94)

This explanation implies that medical rationality, that is using a scientific or biological idiom in the context of the epistemic culture of statistics, is basically relevant, as many other studies based on Foucault have also shown (Rose 2007, Bock von Wülfingen 2007, Knecht 2008). At the same time, this kind of naturalising can obviously complement or even be neutralised by a strategy of supernaturalising based on religious operationalisations, as indicated by social studies on ARTs – and it is a prominent theme in Sarah Franklin's work (1997, 2006). With this strategy of supernaturalisation or sacralisation, I propose to expand Thompson's model.

Thompson calls the affiliation to the Mormon church an 'unusual commodity', which is somewhat strange. Although large parts of the population in the United States and Europe do not explicitly rely on religious reasoning, other parts adhere to these kinds of 'alternative operationalizations' (Thompson 2005: 94), not to mention people in non-Western societies. And referring to Yanagisako and Delaney (1995), we can assume that more Western people, practitioners, patients and third parties alike, do make reference to this religious mode of reasoning if the beginnings of life are at stake. Therefore, it is important that the entanglement of medical and religious reasoning is robustly conceptualised and investigated in social science research of ARTs. This is not yet worked out in detail in Thompson's book, but in a comment on several studies on religion and IVF, she writes that religion plays a productive part in reproductive technologies and that an emphasis on religion 'adds immeasurably to our understanding of reproductive technologies' (Thompson 2006: 560-561).

The social effects of ARTs: conservative or innovative?

Thompson (2005) concludes that innovative reproductive technologies not only strengthen old ways of claiming kinship and gender identity, but also lead to new configurations. She is interested in these 'seeds of change', but also aware of the 'conservative strategies that extend old concepts and understandings' (Thompson 2005: 146). Particularly when male infertility is at stake, male sexual identity is also destabilised, and strategies for the 'management of stigma' (Thompson, 2005: 128) are mobilised – not only by the men concerned but also by medical practitioners and partners. In this context, mostly conservative strategies based on conventional gender scripts come into play. These can be naturalising, if they concern virility in the sense of the quantity or quality of sperm, or they can be socialising strategies, if the potential to be a good father has to be proven. In both cases, stereotypical forms of gender performativity are displayed. Thompson (2005: 143) falls back upon on a somewhat functionalist explanation when she suggests that

> Scripted, performative repertoires of gender in this site function to enable order and normalize innovation, especially innovations in the ontology of sex, gender, and kinship and in their implications for society.

An approach that also takes interests of individual actors and issues of power more into consideration could give subtler answers.

Thompson (2005: 178) considers ARTs as part of 'extended cultural and natural biologies' that enable and influence both innovative ways of affiliation or relatedness and hegemonic reification of old ways of classifying and valuing human beings. Referring to Butler's theory of performativity, Thompson suggests that although ARTs and other forms of biomedicine are in large parts motivated by hegemonic family forms, they also subvert these forms. This tendency has been visible for some time in the United States and Britain in single women and lesbian and gay couples' access to ARTs; but Thompson only focuses on heterosexual couples in her study. Strathern and Franklin, who work on ARTs in Britain, also think that these technologies transform kinship and gender relations, but based on other theoretical assumptions. Strathern argues in many of her publications that the knowledge strategy of making the implicit explicit, meaning the uncovering of assumptions, has a displacement effect, which is an irreversible process (Strathern [1993] 1999, 1995; Franklin [1993] 1999). Strathern (1999: 184, emphasis added) explains this very poignantly in one of the first ethnographic studies on reproductive medicine:

> Everything is new and nothing is new. The paradox posed by the 'implication' of the NRTs dissolves if one realises that *conservation is itself a force for change*. By constantly attempting to make sense of their circumstances, justify their actions, find reasons for their values, Euro-Americans conserve their sense of themselves in creating new contexts out of old ones.

Conclusions

Normalisation could be more clearly conceptualised if it is not defined as a two-layer procedure with different components, as Thompson explains it. I propose a redefinition of normalisation as a process of making identities, subjectivities and social relationships self-evident by means of a diverse spectrum of natural, biological, social and religious idioms or rhetorical strategies, in addition to the use of statistics and routines as general practices (see also de Jong, this volume). Such a definition concurs with approaches of Yanagisako and Delaney, as well as that of Franklin who argue for a unified analysis of science and religion. This means both an expansion and differentiation of Thompson's model, analytically distinguishing the natural from the biological, and adding the sacred as an additional strategic realm of normalising as well as the social. To formulate this more generally, I suggest that we have to make sense of the entanglements of medical and religious rationales in processes of ARTs. This makes the model Thompson proposes more subtle and applicable to a broader range of contexts. Moreover, we should further reflect on what is excluded from normalisation and what remains abnormal in this conceptual frame.

It is important to place more emphasis on issues of power, institutional structures, and subjectivity, especially if we would like to improve our understanding of how ARTs are differently normalised in various social contexts and why the effects of ARTs are conservative in certain contexts, whereas in others they are innovative. For example, why are egg donation and gestational surrogacy allowed in Russia and other countries, but forbidden in Switzerland and Germany? Or why is IVF for singles, lesbians and gays in all three countries still often considered abnormal? I would argue that in processes of ARTs, standardised bodies, forms of personhood and families are produced together with non-standardised ones, which may or may not be suppressed. Further investigations of forces of power, including cosmologies, may explain what remains abnormal for the time being and why making use of ARTs, and thus displacing the boundaries of the body, family, kinship and gender, is in many places still a subject of taboo and secrecy – in Russia, Switzerland and Germany as well.

Notes

[1] The concept of kinning has been developed in more detail with respect to transnational adoption by Signe Howell (2003). By kinning she means 'the process by which a foetus or new-born child (or previously unconnected person) is brought into a significant and permanent relationship with a group of people that is expressed in a kin idiom' (Howell 2003: 465). She considers this a universal process which is, in all societies, related to life cycle rituals that guarantee 'kinned subjectiviation' (Howell, 2003: 466), but which is not necessarily recognised as such.

[2] In later studies, Delaney (2001) investigates the significance of the origin story of Abraham for patriarchal kinship thinking today in Western societies. In an article abut the reconceptualisaion of kinship, she concludes: 'Because biblical notions of kinship are embedded in secular scientific theory, it is difficult to move beyond them. Kinship may be about procreation, but procreation is not just about biology, however conceived. From the beginning, it has incorporated aspects of the divine.' (Delaney 2001: 462).

References

Bharadway, A. (2003) Why adoption is not an option in India: the visibility of infertility, the secrecy of donor insemination, and other cultural complexities, *Social Science and Medicine* 56: 1867-1880.

Bock von Wülfingen, B. (2007) *Genetisierung der Zeugung: Eine Diskurs- und Metaphernanalyse reproduktionsgenetischer Zukünfte.* Bielfeld: transcript.

de Jong, W. (2008) Intimität auf dem Prüfstand: Neue Verwandtschaftsverhältnisse durch assistierte Reproduktionstechnologien, in I. Tomkowiak und W. Egli (Hg) *Intimität.* Zürich: Chronos Verlag: 137-154.

Delaney, C. (2001) Cutting the ties that bind: the sacrifice of Abraham and patriarchal kinship, in S. Franklin and S. Mckinnon (eds.) *Relative Values: Reconfiguring Kinship Studies.* Durham: Duke University Press: 445-467.

Cussins, C. (1987) Producing reproduction: techniques of normalization and naturalization in an infertility clinic, in S. Franklin and H. Ragoné (eds) *Reproducing Reproduction: Kinship, Power and Technological Innovation.* Philadelphia: University of Pennsylvania Press: 66-101.

Franklin, S. ([1993] 1999) Making representations: the parliamentary debate on the human fertilisation and embryology act, in J. Edwards, S. Franklin, E. Hirsch, F. Price and M. Strathern Technologies of Procreation: *Kinship in the Age of Assisted Conception.* London, New York: Routledge: 127-165.

Franklin, S. (1997) *Embodied Progress: A Cultural Account of Assisted Conception.* London, New York: Routledge.

Franklin, S. (2006) Origin stories revisited: IVF as an anthropological project, *Culture, Medicine and Psychiatry* 30: 547-555.

Howell, S. (2003) Kinning: the creation of life trajectories in transnational adoptive families, *Journal of the Royal Anthropological Institute* 9: 465-484.

Inhorn, M.C. (2002) The 'local confronts the 'global': infertile bodies and new reproductive technologies in Egypt, in M.C. Inhorn and F. van Balen (eds) *Infertility Around the Globe: New Thinking on Childlessness, Gender, and Reproductive Technologies.* Berkeley: University of California Press: 263-282.

Knecht, M. (2008) Reproduktionstechnologien und die Biomedikalisierung von Verwandtschaft. Anmerkungen aus ethnographischer Perspektive, *Das Argument* 275: 179-194.

Rose, N. (2007) *The Politics of Life Itself: Biomedicine, Power, and Subjectivity in the Twenty-First Century.* Princeton, Oxford: Princeton University Press.

Schneider, D.M. (1968) *American Kinship: A Cultural Account.* Chicago, London: University of Chicago Press.

Strathern, Marilyn ([1993] 1999) Regulation, substitution and possibility, in J. Edwards, S. Franklin, E. Hirsch, F. Price and M. Strathern *Technologies of Procreation: Kinship in the Age of Assisted Conception.* London, New York: Routledge.171-202.

Strathern, M. (1995) Displacing knowledge: technology and the consequences for kinship, in F.D. Ginzburg, and R. Rapp (eds) *Conceiving the New World Order: The Global Politics of Reproduction.* Berkeley: University of California Press: 346-368.

Strathern, M. (2001) Gender: eine Frage des Vergleichs, in U. Davis-Sulikowski, H. Diemberger, A. Gingrich und J. Helbling (Hg.) *Körper, Religion und Macht: Sozialanthropologie der Geschlechterbeziehungen.* Frankfurt, New York: Campus: 359-393.

Thompson, C. (2005) *Making Parents: The Ontological Choreography of Reproductive Technologies.* Cambridge, Mass.: MIT Press.

Thompson, C. (2006) God is in the details: comparative perspectives on the intertwining of religion and assisted reproductive technologies, *Culture, Medicine and Psychiatry* 30: 557-561.

Yanagisako, S. and C.Delaney (1995) Naturalizing power, in S. Yanagisako and C. Delaney (eds) *Naturalizing Power: Essays in Feminist Cultural Analysis.* London, New York: Routledge: 1-22.

National regimes of reproductive technologies

Assisted reproduction in Russia: legal regulations and public debates

Olga Brednikova, Nadya Nartova, Olga Tkach

In this chapter we aim to provide a background picture of assisted reproductive technologies (ARTs) in Russia. The analytical material is drawn from two national newspapers: *Rossiiskaia Gazeta* (RG), the Russian Newspaper; and *Argumenty i Fakty* (AiF), Arguments and Facts, which publishes state rules and regulations. We begin by outlining the development of in vitro fertilisation (IVF) and other types of assisted reproduction, showing the popularisation of this topic in scientific, medical, and especially public domains. Then we show how, and in what forms, ARTs found their way into legislation.

The popularisation of ARTs: scientifically, medically and publicly

In Russia, ARTs in their contemporary form appeared in the late 1980s. Although these technologies were intensively investigated and tested through experimentation in the USSR, results never went beyond laboratory doors. The births of the first test tube children in 1986[1] were milestones in the development of ARTs in Russia. Since then, artificial insemination and extra corporal fertilisation have become widely publicised and increasingly used medical practices. However, in Russia, these technologies are restricted to infertility treatment. Human cloning, one of the most delicate issues in this area, is prohibited. In 2002, the Federal Law 'On The Temporary Human Cloning Ban' declared a five year moratorium on implementing any new research and conducting experiments with cloning. There is currently public debate, involving politicians, representatives of Russian Orthodox Church, and lay people, about prolonging this moratorium.

There are about fifty clinics that provide ARTs in Russia: thirty in Moscow; six in St. Petersburg; the others in various cities. In 2003, about eleven thousand IVF procedures were carried out across the country.[2] There is an increasing demand each year for such treatments. According to the Ministry of Health, one in six married Russian woman of reproductive age cannot conceive and bear a child without medical intervention.[3] With these figures in mind, two or three times more ART clinics would be needed to serve approximately thirty thousand married couples a year (AiF 26.10.2005). The average age of patients is 34 years (RG 7.7.2006). The success rates for 2003 – 43.1% in St. Petersburg clinics and 32% on average across Russia – were evaluated by Vladislav Korsak, President of the Russian Association of Human Reproduction, as 'relatively high', especially when compared with the European success rate of 27.9 % (AiF 1.11.2006).

The Russian state began to finance ARTs several years ago. Now, IVF treatments can be carried out for free in cases of female infertility; but only one cycle is supported, which is insufficient in practice. Some European states finance reproductive services more extensively. In Finland, for example, three free attempts to conceive are available; in Slovenia, four; and in Belgium, six (AiF 26.10.2005). In Russia, the so-called federal quota of free IVF treatments is limited to 150 couples per year for the whole population. In 2005, St. Petersburg – a city with five million inhabitants – was provided four quotas, but only one patient was able to take advantage of free treatment (AiF 1.11.2006). Moreover, quotas are exclusively distributed between four state clinics: two in Moscow, one in Yekaterinburg, and one in Rostov. Thus, patients from other cities or from rural areas must make long and expensive journeys. Their travel expenses and lodging are not reimbursed. Even if a procedure is formally free, it has costs. Though the Head of the Ministry of Health and Social Development has declared that the government has been considering the possibility of free access to IVF for twenty-five to thirty thousand married couples annually, this idea still does not work.[4]

In order to receive permission for free IVF treatments, it is necessary to obtain a referral from the special Commission of the Ministry of Health and the Russian Academy of Medical Sciences, and to collect a set of health certificates, which requires standing in many different queues for a long time. A common criticism of Russian fertility clinics is that they lack highly skilled staff and financial support. Basically, these technologies are employed in the realm of commercial medicine. Even the seven state-run clinics openly offer ART services on a market basis. It is not accurate to say that wide access is available for ARTs, as these treatments are expensive compared to average salaries in Russia. For the majority of patients, procedures must be paid for out of their own pocket as ARTs are not covered by the state medical insurance. The cost of IVF is relatively high, between sixty to eighty thousand RRUB (2,000-2,500 USD), and half of this expense goes toward medical support of the procedure (AiF 26.10.2005). The price of artificial insemination varies between twenty and thirty thousand RRUB (800-1,000 USD). The cost of a surrogate mother's services frequently depends on real estate prices, which vary considerably in different regions of Russia. As a rule, a surrogate mother obtains from the prospective parents a room, or a one-room apartment, for bearing the baby and giving birth.

The problematic infrastructure of ARTs and the newness of these technologies keep them on the public agenda. Within the last two decades, social attitudes toward the application of these technologies have been gradually changing. In the late 1980s and early 1990s popular science discourse dominated in the media, describing ARTs in metaphorical language such as a 'sacrament of science' or a 'triumph of the human mind' over 'nature's disadvantages' (RG 14.08.1991). Later on, public debate about ARTs became influenced by morality and ethics. Assisted reproduction became mainly negatively valued, and debates about these topics created a moral panic. The mass media, the church, and medical practitioners, as actors in the debate, argued from their specific perspectives, e.g. the topic of surrogacy turned into the problem of baby trafficking. Since motherhood is normative, and nearly obligatory, in Russian culture, issues around reproduction and fertility are highly morally charged. This cultural framing of reproduction and motherhood moves debate about ARTs from the realm of human rights and individual choice, and locates it in the context of cultural problems, demographic crisis and national risks.

The development of ARTs intensified civil activism by both medical doctors and their patients. In St. Petersburg, doctors established an NGO called the 'Russian Association of Human Reproduction'. This organisation focuses on the peculiarities of medical ethics in the practicing of ARTs. The representatives of this group have accumulated political influence because they also participate in public debates as experts on procreation. Consumers of ARTs form another stream of civil activism. A group of female patients created a website called Probirka, which means test tube (www.probirka.ru). Besides spreading important practical information on ARTs, this site serves as a platform for lively debates. More than a thousand visitors discuss urgent social and medical ART problems. The activities of women that resort to the help of reproductive medicine produce a specific alternative communicative space for ART consumers. We define this space as alternative in three ways. First, cyberspace is an alternative to offline communicative communities. Second, this community emerged as a network that contests formal organisational structures of traditional NGOs. Finally, this online community provides a space for solidarity, as opposed to individual consumerist strategies. Participants exchange information, attempt to control doctors' activities and implementation of medical procedures, and support each other emotionally. A recent event initiated by the moderators in cooperation with the magazine *Hochu Rebenka* (I Want to Have a Baby) and the interregional public fund of social solidarity *Nash Vybor* (Our Choice), was the creation of the Crystal Test Tube Award for fertility clinics. The list of clinics nominated for the award was compiled by the visitor's voting results. This example of civil activism by ART consumers reveals the mechanisms of interaction with medical institutions, which were until recently were totally closed against external interventions.

Legal backgrounds of ARTs

The use of ARTs is legally regulated on different levels. Above all, according to the Constitution of Russia (article 38 'State Protection of

Mother and Child') every woman can exercise her right to be a mother. One of the possible ways of securing this right is to make use of 'artificial insemination or embryo implantation'. The legalisation of motherhood and fatherhood while using ARTs is vested in the Family Code of Russia. Details of these rules and their application are provided by the Decree of the Ministry of Health of Russian Federation (2003: No. 67) entitled 'On the use of ARTs in the treatment of female and male infertility'. The main points of this decree and some other laws that have important social outcomes for the use of ARTs are examined below.

Access to the procedures

Clinics and special medical centers are permitted to carry out ART procedures if they possess a state certificate and license according to the 'Legislative basis for the protection of national health' (Ministry of Health of the Russian Federation, 1993: No. 5487-1, article 35). Married couples and single women are welcomed to make use of extra-corporeal fertilization (IVF) and artificial insemination (AI). The usual diagnostic criteria for undergoing IVF and AI with one's husband's sperm is incurable infertility, or if other methods have not worked properly. Besides these medical requirements, conducting AI with a donor's sperm is allowed for a woman who has no sexual partner.

Gynecological, oncological and other diseases can prevent the application of ARTs. Other contraindications are mental diseases, as well as syphilis, HIV, and hepatitis. Preimplantation genetic diagnosis (PGD) is used to detect monogenic and chromosome embryo defects, as well as to determine the sex of an embryo to prevent certain inherited genetic diseases. PGD is used for women with a high risk of giving birth to children with genetic pathologies and is considered an alternative to prenatal diagnosis.

Informed consent is required of all ART patients. Medical centers providing these procedures collect and archive a wide variety of patient data. The Ministry of Health has developed and approved a special questionnaire called 'Individual patient file for the period of ART treatment'. Besides assessments of patient health, this document contains personal information such as passport data, age, nationality, home address, place of work, profession, work position, marital status, and material about the spouse, if it is available.[5]

Biomaterial donations: illegal and permitted

In Russia, donation of sperm and oocytes (undeveloped ova, or eggs) is legal:

> Donors provide their genetic cells to other persons for treating infertility, and do not take up parental duties and responsibility towards a future child. (Ministry of Health of the Russian Federation, 2003: No. 67)

The possibility of twenty births from one donor is the reason for dissolving any agreements with the donor. 'Non-anonymous relatives or acquaintances, or anonymous donors can donate oocytes' (RG 14.08.1991). The donation of oocytes requires informed consent from donors, and is effectuated through the induction of super-ovulation and ovariocentesis. Donors are required to be 20-35 years old, physically healthy, and to have one healthy child.

Donor sperm can be used for both IVF and AI.[6] A sperm donor is required to be 20-40 years old. He should not have 'deviations in normal organometric and phenotypic characteristics' (Ministry of Health of Russian Federation, 2003: No. 67). The documents required by sperm donor programs are: signed informed consent forms; donor questionnaires; individual medical files; and catalogues with descriptions of donors' anthropometric data and phenotypic portraits that are offered to patients. Besides medical data, the questionnaire designed for the donors of sperm and oocytes, like the questionnaire for the patients, also contains social information such as date of birth, address, education, profession, marital status and children.[7] All questionnaires and documents are filled out and coded by medical doctors and are kept in a safe for fifty years. Patients have the right to choose a donor independently and voluntary. Donor catalogues contain detailed description of anthropometric data and phenotypic portrait, but not a donor's profession, bad habits, inherited diseases and sexual preferences.

Embryo donorship is also permitted. Embryo donors can be patients using IVF who have surplus cryo-preserved embryos that are being kept in a bank 'after having obtained a completed family (giving birth to a child)' (Ministry of Health of Russian Federation, 2003: No. 67). The phrase 'completed family' implicitly demonstrates the final goal of the governmental regulation of ARTs, namely the creation of families consisting of a mother, a father, and a child. Based on the voluntary decision and the informed consent of parent donors, these embryos can be used by a childless married couple or single woman. Embryos for donation may also be created as a result of fertilisation of a donor's oocyte with a donor's sperm. According to regulations, patients must be informed that the success rate of using cryo-preserved embryos left over from IVF is lower than that using embryos created from donor gametes. Moreover, recipients should also be provided with phenotypic portraits of the donors. The price of biomaterial for donation is not regulated by law but defined by the clinics and medical centres, according to market demands. The relationship between the clinics implementing ARTs and their patients is regulated by the law 'On Consumer Rights Protection' (amendments of 17.12.1999, 30.12.2001).

Reduction of embryos and fetuses

To prevent obstetric and perinatal complications arising from multiple embryos, legislation allows reduction when three or more embryos are in the womb. Reduction can be implemented on the basis of informed consent from the pregnant woman. Based on a doctor's recommendations, the woman also defines the number of embryos to be reduced. Certain legal rules have been established to control biomaterials: sperm, oocytes and cryo-preserved embryos. These rules mainly cover recording and archiving information on biomaterials,[8] which must be kept for fifty years.

Surrogate motherhood

The principle legal basis for regulating surrogate motherhood is the Decree of the Ministry of Health 'On the use of ARTs in treating female and male infertility' (No. 67, 26.02.2003). According to this document, a married couple and a surrogate mother must provide informed consent to participate in a surrogate motherhood program. Access to this program is restricted to married couples having problems with fertility, and is strictly prohibited for single women. Surrogate mothers are recruited on a voluntary basis. A potential surrogate mother is required to be 20-35 years old, psychologically and physically healthy, and to have her own healthy child. Unlike sperm and oocyte donation programs, which maintain the patient confidentiality of donors, married couples are provided with detailed information on the physical and psychological health of the woman who is hired to bear their baby.

Surrogate motherhood is also regulated in the Family Law of the Russian Federation (articles No. 51 'Registration of a child's parents in the birth registration book' and No. 52 'Contesting fatherhood or motherhood', 29.12.1995), and in the Federal Law 'On Civil Status Acts' (article 16). A child born after the use of surrogacy on the basis of a written agreement has to be regarded as the child of the mother and her husband only if the biological (surrogate) mother does not recognize the child as hers (Family Law of the Russian Federation, Section 4, Chapter 10, article 51). According to the Federal Law on 'Civil Status Acts' (15.11.1997), several documents must be submitted in addition to the birth certificate to register a child born from a surrogate mother. These documents include an official statement from the surrogate that the couple who hired her are the parents of the child. In the event that a surrogate wishes to keep the baby, Russian Family Law protects her rights as the legal mother, as mentioned above. According to article No.16 of the Civil Status Acts, an application for a child's birth registration should be submitted no later than one month after the birth. A surrogate mother must make her decision within this period. As a rule, her written consent should be validated by a medical clinic, usually by a maternity hospital. It is prohibited for both the married couple, who gave their consent for the implantation of their embryo into another woman, and the surrogate mother to contest motherhood and fatherhood after the information about the parents has been filed and written in the birth registration book.

Legislation of surrogate motherhood is ambiguous and contains a number of hidden dangers. A surrogate mother can change her mind and may refuse to register the bio-parents as the child's parents. In this case, she enjoys legal priority as the biological mother. If a surrogate mother wants to keep the baby, she submits papers from the medical clinic where she gave birth, then legally registers herself as the child's mother. The rights of the child's biological parents are not protected under the law. Russian legislation also does not allow any payments for a surrogate mother's service, such contracts are arranged informally. Formal contracts guarantee only the transfer of civil rights and responsibilities from one parent to another.

Another problem with the legislation of surrogate motherhood is that these regulations presuppose the implantation of an embryo conceived through fertilisation of a bio-mother-wife's oocyte by a bio-father-husband's sperm. Other variants of artificial insemination are not covered. For example, the use of donated oocytes or sperm makes the registration of the child extremely complicated. According to this regulatory framing, use of surrogacy is restricted to female infertility. Thus, a fertile woman who does not want to bear a child and give birth, and who would like to delegate this work to another woman, does not receive legal support. Moral and ethical issues around surrogate motherhood have been hotly debated in Russia. There is a threat of commercialisation of surrogacy because of inappropriate legislation and the low living standards of the majority of the population. Therefore, different actors search for possibilities to reduce the commercial dimension of surrogacy, while trying to strengthen its moral component. Recruiting relatives from different generations as surrogate mothers is seen as a means of emphasising mothering and deemphasising commercial relationships. Although the fundamental right of a child to know his or her parents is approved by the Family Law, the applications of ARTs and the various forms of donorship are not yet regulated according to this principle.

Medical ethics

Besides Russian legislation, medical activities for procreative purposes are regulated by professional codes, including international ones. Russian medical doctors signed 'The Declaration on Artificial Insemination and Embryo Transplantation' passed by the 39th World Medical Assembly in 1987 in Madrid. According to this declaration, doctors carrying out ARTs should follow the norms of medical ethics, such as the following:

- '(…) careful attitude to the health of a future mother and embryo from the first days of life (…)'
- Patients and donors should be informed of 'the goal, method, risks, troubles and possible failure of ART treatments'. Consent for participation in the procedure should be 'voluntary and informed'.
- '(…) patients have the right to confidence and protection of privacy, as with any other medical treatment'
- If carrying out IVF results in a surplus of oocytes that are not immediately used for the infertility treatment, the donors should also decide about their disposal. Surplus oocytes can be: a) disposed of, b) cryo-preserved and then kept frozen, or c) fertilised and then cryo-preserved.
- '(…) a doctor cannot neglect his/her moral principles, but should be attentive and respectful with regard to the moral and ethics principles of patients'
- The fertilisation process should not be interfered with to choose a fetus' sex, except for those cases when such interference allows the avoidance of inherited pathologies correlated with sex.[9]

Conclusion

Today the legal status of ARTs in Russia is relatively liberal. Although highly regulated, treatment possibilities – including surrogate motherhood and cryo-preservation of oocytes and embryos – are legally permitted and currently practiced. The only significant restriction to artificial procreation treatments is the priority given to married couples. At the same time, the medical infrastructure is insufficient for physicians and can not meet the increasing demands for fertility treatment. Prospective patients also do not have adequate access to these services. Thus, the implementation of ARTs has become increasingly commercialised, though mechanisms of the market do not work precisely to enhance the situation. Increasing civil activism, initiated both by physicians and consumers of ARTs, brings these problems into public awareness. These topics disappear neither from the media nor from politics, and these debate occur within an overlapping space of medicine, legislation, market and morality, with an emphasis on the last realm.

Notes

[1] They were born one-by-one in the Moscow Centre for Obstetrics, Gynaecology and Perinatology, in February, and in the Academies of Medical Sciences in Leningrad and in the Scientific Research Institute of Gynecology and Obstetrics, in September.

[2] Data on the number of artificial inseminations for the same period are not available.

[3] Statistics on male infertility are not available, perhaps because there is hardly any debate on the reproductive health of men.

[4] These are numbers of 2006. The numbers of IVF cycles and quotas supported by the state are slightly higher in 2009.

[5] Interestingly, this questionnaire presupposes questions on professional health danger and bad habits only for husbands. The last issue refers only to smoking and alcohol abuse, but does not include drug abuse.

[6] The use of anonymous donor sperm is only allowed when frozen or unfrozen sperm had passed two negative HIV, syphilis, and hepatitis tests. The use of frozen or unfrozen sperm prevents transmission of HIV, syphilis, hepatitis, and other infections. It also prevents the possibility of a meeting between the donor and the recipient.

[7] In the questionnaire, sperm and oocyte donors interestingly differ in the phenotypic characteristics section. The male variant contains the following items: height, weight, hair (straight, wavy, curly), hair color, eye shape (European, Asian), eye color (blue, green, grey, brown, black), nose (straight, hogged, snub-nosed, wide), face (round, oval, narrow), forehead (high, low, regular). The female variant includes the following criteria, besides the above mentioned items: build (normal, slender, hyperslender), clothing, foot and breast size.

[8] The Decree No. 67 of the Ministry of Health declares that all medical centers offering ARTs should keep special files: Record of the registration, keeping and using of patients' (and donors') oocytes; Record of the registration, keeping and using of patients' (and donors') sperm; Record of the registration, keeping and using of cryoreserved embryos; Individual files of patients using ARTs; Individual file of sperm (and oocyte) donors; Register of Artificial Insemination Treatments.

[9] http://www.med-pravo.ru/International/IVF.htm/ (last accessed July 22, 2009)

Source material

1. Constitution and law

- Constitution of Russia (article 38 'State Protection of Mother and Child')
- Legislation basis for the protection of national health' (No. 5487-1, article 35, 22.07.93)
- Decree of the Ministry of Health of Russian Federation (No. 67, 26.02.2003) 'On the use of ARTs in the treatment of female and male infertility'
- Family Law of the Russian Federation (articles No. 51 'Registration of a child's parents in the birth registration book' and No. 52 'Contesting fatherhood or motherhood', 29.12.1995)
  Federal Law 'On Civil Status Acts' (article 16)
- Law 'On Consumer Rights Protection' (changes of 17.12.1999, 30.12.2001).

2. Public initiatives

- www.probirka.ru (last accessed July 22, 2009)

3. International convention
- 'The declaration on artificial insemination and embryo transplantation' passed by the 39th World Medical Assembly in 1987 in Madrid.

4. *Rossiiskaia Gazeta* (RG), the Russian Newspaper
- 14.08.1991
- 7.7.2006

5. *Argumenty i Fakty*
- 26.10.2005
- 1.11.2006

Assisted reproduction in Switzerland and Germany: regulative and social contexts

Shahanah Schmid

In this chapter I aim to provide a background picture of assisted reproduction technologies (ARTs) in Switzerland, including a brief look at the situation in Germany. I outline the development of in vitro fertilisation (IVF) and other forms of assisted reproduction in Switzerland, showing both the spread of the medical applications, as well as how, and in what form, they found their way into constitution and law. This account is roughly structured by decades: I start in the experimental 1980s; continue through the decade of legislation and standardisation, the 1990s; and conclude with the developments of the 21st century. I then turn to Germany and discuss the key differences and similarities of the current regulative situation in the two countries.

The experimental 1980s

Soon after the famous birth of Louise Brown in 1978 was made public, fertility specialists around the world attempted to replicate the procedure. In Switzerland, the place and year of the first successful attempt is somewhat contested. The first IVF induced pregnancy is credited to the University Women's Clinic in Basle, in 1982[1] – but sources do not state if this pregnancy resulted in a live birth or not. As a cantonal public referendum declared IVF to be illegal in Basle in 1990, Maeder (1992: 363) does not even list Basle as a place where IVF was practiced. The cantonal fertility clinic of Ticino, based in Locarno, claims the first 'pregnancy and birth' by IVF for itself, in 1984.[2] The first birth of an IVF baby in Zurich, at the University Hospital, is claimed to have been in 1986 by the physician then in charge of establishing reproductive medicine, Dr. Elisabeth Möhr.[3] In that decade, clinics were newly established and procedures were quite experimental still, with low success rates[4] and little regulation. What legislation did exist was not federal, but rather local, varying from canton to canton.[5] On the other hand, the medical profession introduced its own regulations. In 1985, the Swiss Association of Medical Sciences (SAMW) added guidelines about IVF to its existing rules on donor inseminations (SAMW: 1981). In 1990, integrated regulation of ARTs, including inseminations and IVF, replaced the two previous guidelines. These new regulations vary from very restrictive (e.g. no donor gametes at all in IVF) to relatively permissive (e.g. egg donation) from one issue to the next, and leave much responsibility to practitioners, whose duty it is to establish the appropriateness in individual cases of possible treatments. These rules, however non-binding they were, are a good indication of the experimental character of the approach to ARTs in that period.

Numbers for treatment attempts and success rates for the 1990s are hard to come by, as no national standardised statistics were created, and practitioners did not need specific licensing.[6] A newspaper article written by a physician gives an estimate of 0.1-1% of all children born being conceived by donor sperm (Hagmann 1987 quoted in Gross and Honer 1990: 99), and between 0.5-1% of children being conceived by ARTs, which would have been about 350 children per year (Hagmann 1987 quoted in Maeder 1992: 363).

It was against this background that a public initiative[7] launched by the influential critical consumer magazine 'Der Beobachter' started the process of national legislation. The initiative, which was instigated in 1985 and submitted with the required number of signatures in 1987, was framed as being 'against abuses' of reproductive and genetic technologies in humans. It is worth pointing out that the 'Beobachter-Initiative' brought to national attention issues of specifically human biotechnology, whereas agricultural methods had long been established and regulated. But what's good enough for cows (artificial insemination) and plants (genetic selection) is assumed to have deeper implications for humans, and to provide the opportunity for abuse. Thus, the initiative re-iterated and confirmed an at the time yet fragile split between 'green' and 'red' biotechnologies, which has since become so standardised that many commentators forget how strongly the development of human ARTs is rooted in animal husbandry and agriculture (Franklin 2007).

Today we know reproduction and genetics, research and medical application, adult and embryonic tissue as distinctive spheres – at least in Switzerland – each individually regulated in separate parts of the law. In contrast, these domains were still messily mixed up in the 1980s, as can clearly be seen in the 'Beobachter-Initiative'. The federal council provided a counter-proposal in 1992, in favour of which the proposed Beobachter legislation was eventually withdrawn. This counter-proposal limited the scope of regulation to what we might term 'applied medical repro-genetics'. A new constitutional act based upon this proposal was passed in 1993. Sweepingly, it stated that assisted reproduction must always adhere to the principles of protection of human dignity, personality and the family. More precisely, this constitutional act prohibited all genetic manipulations in gametes and embryos; the mixing of human and non-human genetic material; embryo donation and all forms of surrogacy; and commercial transactions of reproductive material.[8] Further, it reduced the acceptable indications for IVF treatment to cases of clear infertility, with the sole exception of cases where IVF was the only chance to avoid the transmission of a serious heritable disease to a potential child. Also, the maximum number of embryos to be developed during IVF treatment was restricted to those that could immediately be used for procreative purposes. Thus, the act is a curious mix of basic principles, quite broad prohibitions, and detailed regulation of when and how ARTs can legally be applied. As the constitutional act is generally restrictive, it is perhaps surprising that donor insemination is not prohibited. This is despite the question of heterologue[9] procedures having been a key issue of the preceding debates, and little accepted in public opinion (Maeder 1992: 370).

The 1990s: debating legislation, routinising treatment

Thanks to the constitutional act, a more legally secure environment for IVF was established. Practitioners now knew that IVF itself, though restricted, would in all likelihood not become illegal. With the advent of national regulation, individual cantons were no longer able to completely prohibit ARTs. At the same time, success rates rose significantly at the beginning of the decade, because of new procedures and protocols, such as: improvements in cryo-preservation and hormonal stimulation techniques (Imthurn, Macas et al. 1992); the introduction of intracytoplasmic sperm injection (ICSI) in the mid-nineties; and, of course, more experienced physicians and lab workers. Intracytoplasmic sperm injection had the additional effect of widening the indication for IVF to male factor infertility, thus increasing the number of patients who might be treated successfully. Further, Maeder (1992: 385) reports a shift in the medical definition of infertility towards the end of the 1980s: where previously a couple had to have failed to achieve a pregnancy within two years in order to be classified as infertile, this term was now reduced to one year. Obviously, this redefinition opens up the scope of reproductive medicine for more people, and sooner. Over all, the improved success rates, legal security, and larger potential patient population created the basis for a rapid increase in the number of ART clinics and a doubling of treatment numbers in the 1990s. Whereas Maeder (1992: 363) mentions six official clinics in 1990, and estimates 350 children born per year, the statistics published by the Swiss Society for Reproductive Medicine (SGRM - FiVNat) for the year 2000 count nearly 2,800 patients treated in 18 different clinics with 855 resulting pregnancies.

Whilst some legal certainty had been established, and treatment was becoming more and more routine, the legislative battles on ARTs remained hotly contested. On the one hand, the groups which had opposed the constitutional act as too permissive – but had lost out in the voting – soon launched a new initiative: 'For human dignity in reproduction'. This initiative aimed to undo the new constitutional act, instead completely prohibiting IVF, allowing only homologue inseminations for treatment of infertility. The government countered that initiative with a proposal for a law on reproductive medicine (FMedG). Consensus on the legal text was reached in parliament in 1997, and in 2000, voters could decide between the initiative and the law, the latter finding a clear majority.

Running up to the parliamentary voting on the law – and again before the public voting – new topics dominated in the debates. First, pre-implantation genetic diagnostics (PGD) featured strongly, with fears of eugenics never far away, especially within the Social Democratic Party. The Christian People's Party also had reservations, related to meddling with divine will as expressed in an individual's genetic make-up. The liberal argument that the prohibition of PGD was absurd, as it would simply punish women who would then have to go through repeated, legal abortions in order to reach the same goals, was thus repudiated. Second, in the matter of egg donation, the liberal argument for gender equality – men can donate sperm, and receive donated sperm when necessary; so the same should be true for women and egg cells – remained a minority position as well. Feminists were more worried about the threatening reduction of women's bodies to egg-producing machines, subject to doctors' and scientists' gaze and grasp. Christian women on the other hand, along with many others, argued against the breaking down of biological motherhood, which had somehow gained sanctity. Whereas the social and the biological mother need obviously not be the same, it was felt that the biological should not be further divided – into a gestational and a genetic mother.

The law, which came into force in 2001, and remains valid, includes the same basic principles and extensive prohibitions as the constitutional act does, with the addition of the principle of child welfare – the welfare of the child-to-be must always have highest priority. But mostly, the new law is a detailed ruling on when, how, by whom, and on whom IVF could be attempted. Today in Switzerland, egg donation and surrogacy remains illegal, whereas sperm donation and use of donor sperm is legal but highly regulated. The law introduced limits as to how often the sperm of one man could be used, and confirms the right of children conceived by donor sperm to know the social identity of their genetic father, at the age of 18. The use of donor sperm is restricted to married couples, whereas all other procedures are open to unmarried couples in stable, long-term relationships.[10] The priority of child welfare is stated to imply that would-be parents must not be too old, and must have the means to provide for a child. Further, the law explicitly prohibits genetic diagnostics on embryos (whereas genetic diagnosis of egg cells remains legal in certain cases). The same is true for preservation: gametes may be preserved, but not embryos. Luckily for IVF patients, embryos are clearly defined by the law as beginning their existence only when the genetic information of the egg and sperm has merged to form a new nucleus. Thus, so called 'pro-nuclei' or 'impregnated eggs' do not fall under this prohibition. The law specifies that at most three such 'pro-nuclei' may be developed to embryos within one treatment cycle. Also, the time in which an embryo is allowed to grow in vitro before being transferred into its mother-to-be's uterus is regulated by this law to be no more than absolutely necessary, before implantation in the uterus becomes medically possible. The law also mandated the creation of a national human bioethics commission to advise parliament on future relevant questions; and requires statistics to be collected and published regularly.[11] Licensing is now required for IVF practitioners, who are also subject to quality controls.

Other than by age, sexuality and to a certain extent, wealth, the law does not restrict access to ARTs. However, clinics' decisions to accept patients are wholly discretionary. In practice, for example, women who are overweight find it difficult to be treated in Switzerland; and some clinics require prospective patients to speak at least one of certain languages with certain fluency in order to avoid misunderstandings. Doctors might also refuse to treat women who appear to them to be mentally unstable. On the other hand, the law that patients must be in a stable (heterosexual) partnership is hard to enforce in practice, as doctors must rely on what patients tell them; and their ability to provide for a child is never questioned, as long as they have the means to pay for the treatment. Over all, it can be observed that the law is very specific. It is no general precaution against abuses of all kinds of new biotechnologies, as the initial 'Beobachter-Initiative' had envisaged. Instead, together with its accompanying ordinance, it provides precise legal regulation for a limited field.

New developments in the 21st century

One important issue originally raised by the 'Beobachter-Initiative' is the matter of research. Parliament had decided early on to split the regulation of medical applications from research and science, and deal with each separately (see for example Rothmayr 2006: 613-614). Thus, once the 'reproductive medicine' bill had passed after more than a decade, the next topic was already waiting. A law related to research on human beings had been promised, but due to perceived urgency,[12] only a law on human embryonic stem cell (hES) research was delivered at first, with the view to later integrate this into more general legislation. In 2004, the Swiss people voted on the new 'Stammzellenforschungsgesetz (StFG)' (law on stem cell research).

This focus on embryonic stem cells meant that, although reproductive medicine had been debated, regulated, debated some more, and finally voted on, it did not disappear from the public stage in the new millennium. Human embryonic stem cell research required human embryos to work with, and where should these come from, if not from IVF?[13]

Although hotly debated in the time before the voting, the proposed stem cell research law (StFG) found a clear majority. A legal paradox ensued. The StFG explicitly allows research on 'surplus' embryos – embryos created during IVF treatment, but not used. On the other hand, in addition to specifying that no embryos may be created for any other reason than for fertility treatments, the FMedG also implicitly prohibits the creation of 'surplus' embryos during such treatment. Short of a woman dying, being diagnosed with cancer, or changing her mind about wanting children in the two days between the actual in-vitro fertilisation and the planned embryo transfer, the intention of the law is that all viable embryos (but not pro-nuclei) created in the laboratory must immediately be 'transferred' to the fertility patients. In summary, a legal grey area remains around the issue of 'surplus' embryos, with one law prohibiting their very existence, and another law allowing stem cell research on them.

Another issue which kept reproductive medicine on the public agenda in the new millennium was the introduction – again by popular voting – of a form of registered civil partnership for homosexual partners. Although the law explicitly excluded partnered couples from fertility medicine, ARTs remained one of the key points of the debates. As the law eventually won a majority in the voting, homosexual couples are now doubly, if not triply excluded from reproductive medicine.[14]

In 2005, Switzerland's first designer baby[15] was born, though obviously conceived outside of Switzerland (Meili and Puntas Bernet 2005). Media interest was huge. At the same time, the liberal party pushed the issue of PGD back onto the legislative agenda. Though similar arguments as in earlier debates were heard, a new issue – disability – played a decisive role. Disability lobbyists were critical towards PGD, arguing that the mere possibility of selecting against disability devalued them as human beings; but in the end it was the personal testimony of one actvist in particular, himself a disabled parliamentarian of the Green party, which turned the tide. Luc Recordon said that if the choice had then been available to his parents, he would rather not have been born at all, than born as he was. After this, the motion to legalise PGD went through, and is now in the process of being adapted into law.

In summary, the 21st century so far has seen a continued public debate on reproductive medicine, through related issues such as hES research; social questioning of who should or should not have children; and a resurgence of questions related to PGD. In the shade of this high public profile of ARTs, practitioners went on with their work. The law – now in force – provides stability and security. Although success rates remained largely stable after reaching 21% pregnancies per treatment cycle in 2001, patient numbers grew steadily and by 2007 had nearly doubled since the beginning of the decade, with 5,481 couples treated in 25 clinics across the country (BFS 2009). This is the unspectacular counterpoint to public outcries and interest in stem cells, PGD and homosexual parents.

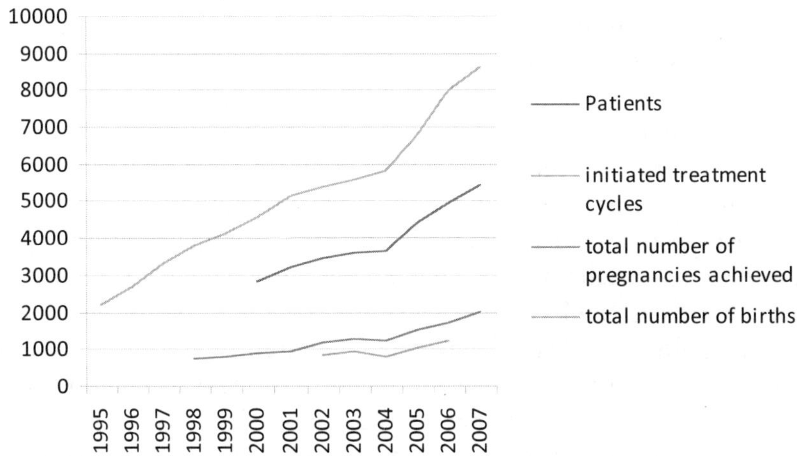

Figure 1: Treatment numbers 1995-2007[16]

The situation in Germany regarding ARTs is similar in many respects, but differs in some key aspects. In vitro fertilisation has been practised for roughly the same amount of time in both countries, with 'Oliver', the first German test tube baby, conceived in 1982 in Erlangen. General principles of what may and may not be practised in fertility treatment were laid down in 1990 in the new 'Embryonenschutzgesetz' (embryo protection law). As in Switzerland, the law prohibits cloning, surrogacy, egg cell donation, and PGD; but it does not regulate those forms of treatment which remain legal. These are instead determined by binding guidelines published by the German medical association (Bundesärztekammer). This might well be the main regulative difference between the two countries. As an effect, medical professionals rather than the public decide on the remaining questions, e.g. those not covered by the law. Although the guidelines are binding – practitioners can be punished and lose their medical licence if they do not adhere to them – there still is more leeway for individual doctors' decisions. In those issues where the medical profession itself is divided, sanctions are not very likely to be pursued; and changes to the guidelines are more frequent and easier to obtain than changes to a law.[17] Yet, by themselves, the guidelines are not considerably more or less conservative than the Swiss legislation. For instance, they equally exclude homosexual partners and single people from ARTs use. In some respects, German medical self-regulation is basically the same as the Swiss law, but leaves slightly more room for interpretation. For heterologue treatments, the guidelines state that they should be practised with unmarried partners 'only under very careful consideration'; and they also recommend embryos not to be cryo-conserved 'except in extreme circumstances'. One potentially far-reaching difference between the Swiss and German situations concerns sperm donor anonymity. Unlike in Switzerland, donor children in Germany have the right to claim not just knowledge of, but also legal parenthood rights from their donor genetic father. This seriously restricts the number of willing donors. However, as ICSI has developed into the treatment of choice for male factor infertility, usage of donor sperm is increasingly rare in all contexts, not just where donor anonymity and legal protection is lacking.

Some considerable social conservatism can be made out in the way health insurance covering ARTs is regulated in Germany. Since a general reform in 2004, insurance covers 50% of the costs of up to three cycles of IVF treatment;[18] but cover is restricted to clearly defined groups. In order to claim these expenses, patients must be married, not use donor sperm, be between 25 and 40 (women) or 50 (men) years old, and undergo independent counselling before they start treatment. As a result of these restrictions, many potential patients must cover the costs themselves.

Germany's example clearly illustrates that the way ARTs are financed has strong effects on treatment uptake. When financing changed from 100% to 50% coverage, new treatments dropped dramatically, from approximately thirty-three thousand in 2003 to approximately seventeen thousand in 2004 – less than in 1997. Since then, the numbers have only slightly recovered, with approximately twenty-two thousand new first treatments in 2007, which is about the same level as in 1999. In contrast to Switzerland, where treatment numbers nearly doubled every decade (see above), the changes in health insurance regulation caused a massive setback in Germany.

Conclusion

We started this overview in the 1980s, when IVF was first attempted in Swiss and German clinics. This could be dubbed the experimental decade. Not only were the procedures still new and usually unsuccessful, but regulation of these procedures was also tentative; medical associations attempting self-regulation, and policy makers testing the waters for what degree of permissiveness and restriction could be capable of gaining a majority. In Switzerland, the following decade saw the introduction of the constitutional act and the law on reproductive medicine, both passing public votes. Accordingly, emphasis lay on negotiation and debate, both in parliament and in public in the 1990s. In this decade, opinions were formed, became firm, and were written into legislation. Today, the legal situation regarding ARTs in Switzerland is very restrictive socially, but less so from a medical point of view: Although highly regulated, treatment possibilities as they are currently practised around the world are not significantly limited, with the exception of egg donation and surrogacy. With the growing experience of the physicians along with increasing treatment numbers, IVF began to gain the quality of routine, if not precisely normality. Finally, after the turn of the millennium, the legal framework provided a stable background on which ARTs prospered. The topic did not disappear from the media nor from politics, however; on the contrary, public awareness remained high and differentiated.

Notes

[1] See for example an article based on an interview with the physicians involved at the time, on the website of the self-help organisation 'Verein Kinderwunsch': http://www.kinderwunsch.ch/literat/wewo2-d.cfm (last accessed May 19, 2009), and a newspaper article on the clinic's 100 years anniversary (Jenny 1996).

[2] See http://centro-fertilita.eoc.ch/centro-fertilita/_eng/chisiamo/storia.asp (last accessed May 19, 2009). However, in a portrait of the clinic published as a series in a Swiss fertility journal, the authors claim the same event to have taken place in 1983 (Krämer and Stamm 2004). Perhaps the conception was achieved in 83, but the baby was born in 84.

[3] http://www.gynart.ch/index.php?id=30 (last accessed May 19, 2009)

[4] Imthurn et al. (1992) report a clinical pregnancy rate of 6% per punctuation until 1988, improving to 35% in 1991. This increase is mainly attributed to the introduction of a new ovary stimulation protocol and improved cryopreservation techniques.

[5] Rothmayr (2006: 598) declares that 10 out of 26 cantons had state rulings on ARTs in the 1980s, that were subject to legal challenges in the courts (Rothmayr 2006: 607)

[6] Maeder (1992: 387) mentions a science journalist who failed to extract any meaningful numbers from the SAMW, despite their claim to be collecting statistics.

[7] In Switzerland, a public initiative aims at changing the constitution. If enough signatures in support of the initiative can be gathered, parliament is required to submit it to a general public voting; though they do have the option of presenting a counter-suggestion alongside it.

[8] As part of the general revision of the constitution, a new clause was included in the year 2000, which specifically prohibits cloning.

[9] Heterologue, as opposed to homologue, means involvement of donor gametes.

[10] Treatment is restricted to heterosexual couples, as eligible couples must fulfil the conditions necessary to become mother and father as stated in the civil code.

[11] However, although this was made law in 2001, the first official statistics were published in 2006, covering the 2003-2005 period. Before that, FiVNat published yearly statistical reports.

[12] Scientists and funders had pushed research onwards.

[13] See Franklin (2006) for more on the connections between IVF and embryonic stem cells.

[14] First, the civil code states that a person can only become a mother by giving birth, thus making the existence of any form of 'second mother' impossible. Second, the FMedG states that ARTs may only be provided for couples who can legally become parents, referring to the civil code; and by prohibiting surrogacy, it restricts gay couples' access to ARTs. And third, the law on registered homosexual partnerships explicitly prohibits adoption as well as access to ARTs.

[15] Also known as 'saviour baby' or 'bébé médécine'; a child conceived and selected by PGD in vitro to save a sick older sibling by donating umbilical stem cells, bone marrow or other tissue.

[16] Numbers are derived from the yearly published FiVNat-reports (1995-2001) and the Federal Bureau for Statistics reports (2002-2007). The latter include all Swiss IVF clinics, the former only members – but there is only one clinic which is not a member.

[17] In contrast, the Swiss medical self-regulation statements from the 1980s and 1990 have since not been updated, as they have been superseded by the law.

[18] Before 2004, insurance covered 100% of the costs.

Source material

1. Constitution and law

- Bundesverfassung der Schweizerischen Eidgenossenschaft vom 18. April 1999, Art. 119 (Fortpflanzungsmedizin und Gentechnologie im Humanbereich, S. 35)
- Bundesverfassung der Schweizerischen Eidgenossenschaft vom 29. Mai 1874, Art. 24novies (S. 10-11)
- SR211.231 Bundesgesetz vom 18. Juni 2004 über die eingetragene Partnerschaft gleichgeschlechtlicher Paare (Partnerschaftsgesetz, PartG)
- SR810.11 Bundesgesetz vom 18. Dezember 1998 über die medizinisch unterstützte Fortpflanzung (Fortpflanzungsmedizingesetz, FMedG)
- SR810.110.2 Fortpflanzungsmedizinverordnung vom 4. Dezember 2000 (FMedV)
- SR810.31 Bundesgesetz vom 19. Dezember 2003 über die Forschung an embryonalen Stammzellen (Stammzellenforschungsgesetz, StFG)

2. Public Initiatives

- Eidgenössische Volksinitiative 'gegen Missbräuche der Fortpflanzungs- und Gentechnologie beim Menschen' ('Beobachter-Initiative') http://www.admin.ch/ch/d/pore/vi/vis182t.html (last accessed May 19, 2009)

- Eidgenössische Volksinitiative 'zum Schutze des Menschen vor Manipulationen in der Fortpflanzungstechnologie (Initiative für menschenwürdige Fortpflanzung [FMF])' http://www.admin.ch/ch/d/pore/vi/vis241t.html (last accessed May 19, 2009)

3. Parliamentary debates
   Amtliches Bulletin - Die Wortprotokolle von Nationalrat und Ständerat:
- Nationalrat - Sommersession 2005 - Fünfzehnte Sitzung - 16.06.05-15h00
- Nationalrat - Sommersession 1998 - Zehnte Sitzung - 22.06.98-14h30
- Nationalrat - Sommersession 1998 - Elfte Sitzung - 23.06.98-08h00
- Nationalrat - Sommersession 1998 - Dreizehnte Sitzung - 24.06.98-15h00
- Nationalrat - Sommersession 1998 - Vierzehnte Sitzung - 25.06.98-08h00
- Nationalrat - Wintersession 1998 - Vierte Sitzung - 03.12.98-08h00
- Nationalrat - Wintersession 1998 - Fünfzehnte Sitzung - 18.12.98-08h00

4. Swiss Association of Medical Sciences (SAMW)
- Medizinisch-ethische Richtlinien für die artifizielle Insemination, SAMW 1981, Basel
- Medizinisch-ethische Richtlinien für die in vitro Fertilisation und den Embryotransfer zur Behandlung der menschlichen Infertilität, SAMW 1985, Basel
- Medizinisch-ethische Richtlinien für ärztlich assistierte Fortpflanzung, SAMW 1990, Basel

5. German sources
- Deutsches IVF Register, 2008: D.I.R.-Jahrbuch 2007 http://www.meb.uni-bonn.de/frauen/DIR_downloads/dirjahrbuch2007.pdf (last accessed July 3, 2009)
- Bundesärztekammer, 2006: (Muster-)Richtlinie zur Durchführung der assistierten Reproduktion, Novelle 2006. http://www.bundesaerztekammer.de/downloads/AssRepro.pdf (last accessed July 3, 2009)
- Gesetz zum Schutz von Embryonen (ESchG), Ausfertigungsdatum 13.12. 1990
- Sozialgesetzbuch (5. Buch), Paragraph 27a 'künstliche Befruchtung'

References

Bundesamt für Statistik (BFS (2009) Medizinisch unterstützte Fortpflanzung, *BFS Aktuell 14: Gesundheit,* http://www.bfs.admin.ch/bfs/portal/de/ index/themen/14/02/03/key/02.html (last accessed July 17, 2009).

Franklin, S. (2006) Embryonic economies: the double reproductive value of stem cells, *BioSocieties*, 1: 71-90.

Franklin, S. (2007) *Dolly Mixtures: The Remaking of Genealogy* Durham: Duke University Press.

Gross, P. and Honer, A. (1990) Multiple Elternschaften: Neue Reproduktionstechnologien, Individualisierungsprozesse und die Veränderung von Familienkonstellationen, *Soziale Welt*, 41(1): 97-116.

Imthurn, B., Macas, E. et al. (1992) In-vitro fertilization: progress in a method of sterility treatment, *Schweizerische Medizinische Wochenschrift*,122(41): 1509-1516.

Jenny, E. (1996) Ein Ort der Pioniere: 100 Jahre Frauenspital Basel, *Neue Zürcher Zeitung*, 22.08.1996: 17.

Krämer, O. and Stamm, J. (2004) Kantonales Sterilitätszentrum des Tessins in Locarno, *Journal für Fertilität und Reproduktion*, (2): 26-27.

Maeder, C. (1992) Reproduktionsmedizin in der Schweiz: Ergebnisse und Interpretationen einer repräsentativen Bevölkerungsbefragung, *Schweizerische Zeitschrift für Soziologie*, 18(2): 363-391.

Meili, M. and Puntas Bernet, D. (2005) Im Reagenzglas gezeugt, um den Bruder zu retten, *NZZ am Sonntag*, 29. Mai 2005: 28-29.

Rothmayr, C. (2006) Explaining restrictive ART policies in Switzerland and Germany: similar processes – similar results? *German Policy Studies* 3(4): 595-647.

Reproductive technologies, bodies and gender

Surrogate motherhood and sperm donorship in the Russian media: normalising the body

Nadya Nartova

In vitro fertilisation (IVF), as one of the main procedures of assisted reproductive technologies (ARTs), was once an innovative scientific breakthrough, but today it is a widespread practice. Nevertheless, IVF and other ART procedures are still highly problematic because they introduce new types of practices and subjects that have to be included into the common cultural context. As the development of ARTs were not followed by a man-made revolution, or drastic changes to society, we must examine how these practices have been normalised. Charis Thompson (formerly Cussins) defines normalisation as the way in which new information and practices are incorporated into extant procedures and into the already recognized objects of the fertility clinic (Cussins 1998: 67). However, a wider understanding of the concept is necessary. I propose that the concept be broadened and defined as a process whereby new practices are inscribed and legitimised within the existing social order. Discursive strategies of normalisation include both speech and practices, according to Foucault (1996). With this in mind, new practices, subjects and types of connections need to be problematised, defined, explained, justified and re-defined. Moreover, the way in which these new subjectivities and practices are inscribed into existing codes should be examined. The body is one of the main spaces within which discursive and technological debates about ARTs are taking place. Foucault (2002:162) indicates that the body in modern culture is the center of power and power discourses, and it is through the body that subjects are formed. Thus, investigating the body being constructed within ART discourse enables us to understand the normalisation of new practices and forms of corporeality in addition to emerging types of subjects.

In the Russian press two key topics are most acute and problematic in discussions of ARTs: sperm donation and surrogate motherhood.

Although, from a technological perspective, sperm donation and surrogate motherhood are not equivalent procedures, they have become the main representatives of reproductive technologies in Russian discourse, as well as in new visions of the reproductive body. Sperm donation and surrogate pregnancies introduce third parties – in addition to mothers or parents – into the process of impregnation and pregnancy, and are the most acute and indefinite in the social context (Landau and Blyth 1988: 266-267). Sperm donation as a male practice and surrogate motherhood as a female practice constitute and normalise the male and female body for male and female subjects respectively. In this research, I examine how male and female bodies are constituted in ART debates and what kinds of subjects these discourses produce, that is to say how new types of bodies, engendered by new reproductive technologies, are normalized. The data include all publications related to ARTs, between 1996 and 2006, from two Russian periodicals: *Rossiyskaya Gazeta* (RG), Russian Newspaper; and *Argumenty i Fakty* (AiF), Arguments and Facts. Print media discourses are a special type of everyday communication, the analysis of which allows us to reconstruct dominant legitimate representations and contexts, in this case, ones related to ARTs. For discourse analysis of these materials I used the method developed by Harvey Sacks and David Silverman, which is widely used in Russian sociology (Zdrvomyslova and Temkina 2002).

In this article I begin by reviewing the main modes in which bodies are produced and reproduced in media discourses of ART. Then, I will analyse the extent to which surrogate motherhood and sperm donation have been legitimised. Finally, I will review how bodies are produced and normalised in the context of the only morally approved way of surrogate and donorship programs use, that is to say within a reproductive strategy.

General tendencies of body production in print media discourse on ARTs

When studying the production of bodies in ART discourse, it is crucial to mention several important strategies or tropes of constituting the body which are closely related to how bodies are produced in the modern world of medical technology. Further, these tropes are used to make the reproductive body a specially controlled space. The first thing I would like to accentuate is public representation of the reproductive body. In the clinical view, the advanced state of medical monitoring technologies makes the body infinitely open to examination, unwrapping it from the inside. Clinical and technological inspection, with the help of medical vocabulary, make a reproductive body primarily a body of reproductive viscera and their functioning, a body of reproductive processes. No other bodies, no other problematic topics, are described in the Russian mass media in such detail. A reproductive body is not restricted by a specific medical discourse between a patient and a doctor anymore. It has become a body of public knowledge and discourse. Newspaper articles one after another amply describe reproductive organs, their pathologies, impregnation technologies, and so on:

> Taking into account practice in other parts of the world, as well as our own medical experience, the gynaecologists from our clinic developed an exclusive method of treating fallopian tube infertility by endo-video-surgical methods. It is more difficult to treat endocrine infertility as it originates from general abnormal hypothalamus, hypophysis, ovary and uterus functioning, leading to emmeniopathy and dysmaturity of oocyte. (AiF 27.9.2000)

Desacralisation and a technological vision of impregnation make the reproductive body a publicly represented body. Through these discourses, ARTs are normalised in public space.

The second important path in discursive production of the body is the autonomous character of impregnation and the constitution of the body as a service-provider. Visualisation and public representation of impregnation with technological medical vocabularies takes impregnation outside the body. Extensive discussion of germ cells and the organs that produce them, as well as of processes involving these cells, intensifies this re-locating of impregnation. Furthermore, reproduction is represented as a process that occurs on its own, not for the body or the individual, or even inside the body or inside the individual. Cells and embryos exist and function separately from the body, and the body is only serving them:

> After fertilisation an ovum starts dividing and in 2-3 days an embryo with the size of one quarter of a half millimeter in diameter is transplanted into a womb. On day 5 or 6 the embryo 'plunges' into the mucus membrane and further develops in a natural way. (AiF 19.3.1997)

Fertilisation and embryos acquire the status of autonomous subjects. They become the focus, the center of vision and action, while the body merely serves these new subjects.

A third important dimension and effect of the discursive production of the reproductive body that needs to be mentioned is its pathologisation. The normalisation of ARTs is connected to the pathologisation of the reproductive body because it is necessary to explain why, and as a result of which dysfunctions, reproduction does not occur by itself. The reproductive body is thus depicted as a body of sick organs, deformed tissues and impaired processes. A reproductive body is no longer normative, but pathological. Moreover, public visualisation and pathologisation of reproductive bodies occurs within a panopticon of the female body:

> As a surgeon, I am worried a lot about our patients who have undergone surgeries for hystermyoma, endometriosis or genital lesions. Only each 3rd or 4th patient will be able to become pregnant in a natural way, others may become candidates for IVF. (RG 7.7.2006)

In Russian mass media discussions of ARTs, the reproductive body becomes a body of reproductive organs and processes that are publicly watched and monitored. Called upon to overcome dysfunctional body impregnation, ARTs are normalised through descriptions of technologies of visualisation, through public scrutiny and, consequently, through knowledge and control of IVF processes and procedures. The female body is no longer a mother's body, nor a body in the general sense, but an abstract, pathologised and deconstructed body, limited to fertilisation and serving the embryo.

The body and reproductive practices of surrogate motherhood and sperm donorship

The discursive modes of producing the reproductive body that were outlined above generate different problematic body aspects and practices within the field of ARTs. Two of the most vigorously discussed issues around ARTs in the Russian mass media are surrogate motherhood and sperm donation. Obviously, egg donation is closer to sperm donation than surrogacy; but in the material collected, the former is not a contested practice. To be more precise, sperm donation and surrogate motherhood are the most vivid subjects for journalists, and the most difficult from an everyday moral viewpoint. These practices are discussed in Russian newspapers with reference to three key categories: technological developments and cloning; reproductive strategies and practices; and the reproductive body, fertilisation and the commercialisation of pregnancy. These three categories form a moral continuum, within which legitimate and illegitimate practices of using surrogate motherhood and donor sperm are defined. From the perspectives provided in Russian media, the only legitimate, normal and morally approved uses of surrogate motherhood and donor sperm are those related to overcoming infertility. These positive uses lie between cloning and the commercialisation of pregnancy, which constitute the negative poles of the moral continuum, setting the limits of tolerance for the use of ARTs.

In mass media discourses of cloning and the commercialisation of reproduction, surrogate motherhood and sperm donation are represented as sources of biological material for laboratory experiments and for market use. However, these practices are problematic because a human individual cannot be thought of as an anonymous body serving others' pragmatic and ambitious goals. Contemporary cultural codes in Russia do not allow the use of the reproductive body outside the immediate goal of reproduction. Cloning and commercialisation are the designated limits for the use of ARTs, within which acceptable practices of surrogate motherhood and donation are legitimised only as a reproductive strategies for overcoming infertility and giving birth to a child.

Although surrogacy and sperm donation have the right to exist within the Russian cultural framing of ART debates, in everyday life and speech these are relatively new practices. They are controversial and represent ambiguity with respect to subjectivity, corporeality, and family and kinship. Thus, these practices require strong normalisation efforts. It is through the production of a separate body, its definition and redefinition in mass media discourses, that not only the practices of surrogate motherhood and sperm donation are normalised, but also the subjects involved in these programs. Female and male bodies in surrogate motherhood and sperm donation discussions are constituted through the following key topics: body skills, body boundaries, body effects and body outcomes, as well as body money. Here I will trace the contents of these topics related to the kinds of bodies and subjects that are produced and affirmed.

Body skills, body quality and control structures

In ART debates, both male donation and female surrogacy are presented as body skills that are applied to achieve impregnation, pregnancy and childbirth. If a certain individual body is incapable of following the whole reproduction cycle, ARTs facilitate the use of other bodies' reproductive skills. Thus, sperm production and the ability to successfully complete a pregnancy become body skills that are formulated with regard to issues of body quality and control structures, as well as through body and donorship techniques.

Male donorship is described through the conformity of a donor's body to physical, psychological and intellectual health norms that are qualified and confirmed by physicians:

> Only healthy men, according to all medical parameters, can become donors. All their relatives, including grandmothers and grandfathers, are checked. Special attention is paid to donor's psychological health. (RG 27.09.2002)

A donor has to pass numerous tests, including intelligence tests, and has to undergo clinical examination to prove normality:

> It is worth mentioning that the requirements are not limited to impeccable health. The candidate should be good-looking, have some higher education and not be registered with a psychiatrist or substance abuse therapist. (RG 16.12.2003)

Thus, the donor's body qualification resembles that of a model male body. Moreover, it must be proven by experts and test systems.

Female surrogate motherhood also requires physical and mental health qualifications that must be proved by medical experts. This is rarely said, though, and is relegated to the context of medical documentation. The main qualifications of a female surrogate body are moral and cultural characteristics, chosen in accordance with the preferences of the genetic parents. They get acquainted with the surrogate mother and study her biography, her lifestyle and her individual characteristics:

> It took me and my husband quite a long time to choose the future mother for our children. At the institute we were introduced to several women. But they didn't seem trustworthy to us. They were asking for too much money for their services, and it seemed to us that they would care more for their pockets than for our children. And Olga was not from the institute at all. She is an old acquaintance of mine, though not a very close one. I have known her for many years, she has two children, and I have seen her attitude to them. So I had no doubts that she would carry my children in good faith. (RG 8.6.2002)

In this case appropriate surrogate mother is also defined through categories such as responsibility, care, modesty, and attention. A surrogate female body is a caring, moral subject. In sperm donation and surrogate motherhood debates, idealised models exist of a qualified male body, assessed by medical experts; and a caring female body, which is confirmed and constituted by an acceptable way of life as judged by genetic parents.

Body and donation techniques

Sperm donation and female surrogate motherhood are constituted through body techniques that donors and surrogate mothers have to master to participate in donation and surrogate motherhood programs, that is for an efficient implementation of their body skills. Male sperm donation is described in terms of restriction and discipline, because for the production of high quality sperm it is necessary to control and restrain one's body:

> The thing is that a donor should abstain from sex and alcohol for four days prior to ejaculate delivery (…), and the donor should get enough sleep as this affects sperm cell concentration and versatility. (AiF 8.12.1999)

Female surrogate motherhood is constituted through an extension and development of one's own childbearing and motherhood experience. A surrogate mother must have her own children; this is a legal requirement, as it gives her an experience of pregnancy and childbirth. She must also have experience taking care of an embryo and her own body during the phases of pregnancy and childcare. This gives her the necessary skills of care and responsibility that she can apply to the care of the baby:

> So it is better if a surrogate mother is a woman who has her own children, who knows the feelings connected to pregnancy, knows what the act of delivery is, and who has her children and gives them her motherly love. (AiF 15.11.2000)

Male donorship is thus combined with body control and discipline, and surrogate motherhood with an extension of body experience.

Both sperm donation and surrogate motherhood are included into donorship realisation techniques. The sperm delivery process is described as quasi-private. It is performed in a closed room, by way of masturbation, alone. To describe the donation process euphemisms and metaphors are used, a covering and hovering language. The donor's body is left within the private space of familiar practices; it is sequestered from the public eye and external intervention:

> The process of material delivery won't win you by its novelty: alone, still and quiet. A cozy couch in a room, special magazines on the table and a TV set with videocassettes. (AiF 15.6.2004)

In contrast to sperm donation, the process of IVF and the pregnancy of a surrogate mother involve public monitoring of the procedure and processes, and public description. It may involve different fertilisation techniques and attracts numerous specialists. Physicians and genetic parents endlessly control the pregnant body:

> An ovum is taken from a woman by surgery, it is placed into a special medium and given to the laboratory through a special window. It takes the ovum 3-4 hours to adapt to the new environment. If all goes well – and it is watched under a microscope – sperm cells are added to this medium. An embryo in a small transparent glass – it is called a petri dish – is placed into an incubator that looks like an ordinary fridge. Behind the incubator door there are trays where dishes with embryos are kept. Each dish is labelled with the embryo owner's name and the incubator doors are marked as well. Specialists keep a close eye on fertilised cells. The fact of fertilisation alone is not enough, after all. The fertilised cell should start dividing. Only 36, and sometimes even 48 hours later the embryo is transplanted into a womb. (…) Just imagine what kind of devices, instruments and specimen are required for this process! How fine the mastery of medics! (RG 9.1.1998)

A surrogate's body is uncovered, it is public and manipulated by many people. It is placed into monitored spaces of clinical offices and laboratories, while male donation techniques are shielded and quasi-private.

We can say that the articulation of body skills required for sperm donation and surrogate motherhood constitute two different regimens. Male donation is presented as an expert qualification of a model male body and has to do with body discipline; but the donation itself is placed in a quite closed space. The normative female surrogate body, however, is constructed through the prolonged skills of pregnancy, delivery, mothercare experience and adequate behaviour that is primarily assessed by genetic parents. The fertilisation procedure and the pregnancy are located in medical offices for expert monitoring, and are thus displayed in an open space.

Body boundaries, effects and outcomes

In the context of sperm donation and surrogate motherhood, body boundaries are redefined. Male sperm donation involves a widening and dispersion of the donor's body, and extraction of its some parts from the physical donor's body. The donor's sperm is separated from the donor, placed into a special receptacle, and then into a cryo-capsule:

> Received material is collected into a large sterile vial, sorted, purified of related substances and frozen, left to be called for. (AiF 15.6.2004)

Donated sperm becomes an autonomous entity. It undergoes special medical control and manipulation, especially with respect to purification. Furthermore, it is stored separately and used autonomously. Redefinition of female body boundaries with surrogate motherhood involves setting local boundaries within the body and constitutes the surrogate body itself as a boundary. A surrogate mother's body is divided inside, between her own body and the fetal body. They are interconnected, but autonomous spaces. The fetus does not belong genetically to the surrogate mother and is not an extension of her, thus it has to be removed and separated:

> At the moment she is going to become a mother, moreover a mother of twins. The ultra-sound examination shows a boy and a girl that are being carried for her by a different woman – Olga. 'Aren't you confused by the fact that these are not properly 'your' children?' I asked Tatyana. 'What do you mean, 'not mine'? They developed out of my cells. In my opinion, rather than lamenting your whole life about having no children, it is better to seek for a surrogate mother's help. Besides, they told us that the children will look after us and will inherit all our characteristic features.' (RG 8.6.2002)

A surrogate mother's body becomes a living boundary, as it separates genetic parents from the child and involves different control systems – from the side of physicians, genetic parents and her own control. Her body is a crossover point of different interests and manipulations that are revealed here:

> Olga decided to become a surrogate mother for the sake of her son. The five-year-old Andryushka needs to undergo an operation, and there is no other way in Tver region to earn ten thousand dollars. Customers from Moscow were found. A contract was signed, a baby was 'lodged'. And then the nightmare started. First those people from Moscow requested that she moves to an ecologically safer region. Moreover, she had to go without Andryushka as he could infect the 'babycarrier' with rubella. A special supervisor was hired to read her poetry, make her listen to classical music including Bach and take for three-hour walks, in sun or rain. If Olga fell ill, she was not allowed to take pills, to avoid harm to the future child. She was also not allowed to touch her belly, to avoid making the baby accustomed to his hired mother. (AiF 25.2.2004)

The sperm donor's body, though it is widened and dispersed when sperm is taken beyond its boundaries, still keeps its integrity. At the same time, the female surrogate body becomes problematic because numerous boundaries are defined, redefined and fought for within it.

With sperm donation and surrogate motherhood, different body effects are produced, and different bodily outcomes are achieved. Male donation is presented as painless, not connected to loss, as situational and a short manipulation of the body – one delivers sperm and forgets about it. Donation qualifies a male body as a model body, and is connected for this body neither with loss, nor with memories or with an experience prolonged in time:

> In comparison to blood donation, there is absolutely no loss in this process, only pure pleasure. (AiF 26.10.2005)

A donor's body is a body that keeps its integrity. It is not connected to the offspring, as anonymity is guaranteed to the donor and his private responsibility is excluded. For the male donor's body there are no children as a result of his body. He will never see or know them:

> For our patients the donors are fully anonymous. Pictures that are often requested are out of question. Similarly, the donors do not have the right to know who used their sperm. (AiF 19.3.97)

A female body during surrogate motherhood is constituted as traumatised, burdened by the pregnancy and the experience of delivery. It is a body influenced by a long pregnancy period, a painful delivery, complications and consequences after the act of delivery. This is a body losing its integrity and quality, losing its health and wearing out:

> It is also possible to name a sum of money necessary for the rehabilitation of a surrogate mother after the act of delivery and for the treatment of possible complications connected to the pregnancy and the delivery. (RG 21.2.2006)

Moreover, the surrogate mother is left without the baby, which was once so intimate and familiar to her body:

> None of my friends can understand, how one can give away or sell a baby that one has born. (AiF 25.2.2004)

The other possibility is that the surrogate mother is left with the baby, in the event that its genetic parents refuse to accept it. This is a forced continuation of what was a voluntary experience. For the surrogate mother, surrogacy is always a story to be continued, with the possibility of loss or forced acquisition. From this analysis we can conclude that sperm donorship is constituted as an anonymous painless action without consequences, while surrogate motherhood is a realm of great uncertainty with regard to results, complications, decisions and situations.

Body money

Both male donations and surrogate motherhood are associated with monetary rewards; but this market service-money exchange is legitimised and represented in different ways and has a different status for a male and a female subject. Male donorship is paid for, that is to say patients pay for a sperm 'dose'. This was stated in each article and was represented as legitimate, earned income:

> For more than two years already Andrey F. has earned extra income from being a sperm donor: 2-3 times per week he delivers sperm to the cryobank of a medical center. Actually, Andrey is working as a bodyguard in a sales company, and the idea of starting an additional business was suggested to him by a friend (…). (AiF 8.12.1999)

As a donor, a man is selling his body skills and fairly receives money for that. His body is qualified as a model male body (he is a real man!) and the cultural code prompts him to earn money. In both contexts this is done by using body skills.

In contrast female surrogate motherhood is constituted as a non-monetary exchange, as childbirth (pregnancy and the act of delivery) cannot be adjusted to the market structure – they have to be altruistic. A surrogate mother is a relative or an acquaintance having free will to help a childless couple and carries and gives birth to a child:

> Mother gave birth to the twins for a childless sister. She officially became a surrogate mother to help her relative and to solve her financial problems as she is bringing up two children alone. Her sister and her husband are wealthy people but do not have children. (RG 21.2.2006)

A surrogate mother is a woman who invests received money into her own children, their treatments or sustenance, quasi-for-free, showing her altruism in regard to her own children:

> 'When I was offered the chance to be a surrogate mother,' Olga says, 'I was at a loss. I had never heard of that before. (…) Of course, I did it for money. I am bringing up two children alone and with my income as a layout designer, that is not easy. So after brief a consideration, I decided to accept the offer of the childless couple.' (RG 8.6.2002)

Thus, surrogate motherhood is designated and constituted as a moral action of assistance to a childless couple and her own children, but not as income. This money could not be spent for her own desires or a new fur coat. Female reproductive body skills do not have a monetary equivalent, and cannot be a legitimate income. Surrogacy is a moral action, a resource for investments into others, altruism. In sum, men's use of body skills is considered a legitimate income, while surrogate motherhood is banned from such commercialisation.

Having reviewed the key points – body skills, body boundaries, body effects and body outcomes and body money – we can say that sperm donation and surrogate motherhood produce two different types of bodies and two different subjects. A sperm donor is an almost ideal man with a model body who earns money by his body skills as a man should. A male body is kept integral and private, including anonymity. It is not damaged either by unforeseen consequences or by a prolonged experience, pain or loss. A surrogate mother's body, in contrast, needs constant control and monitoring, which are overt and public. It is constantly manipulated and undergoes procedures. It is fragmented and problematic, with internal boundaries. It wears out, it experiences loss and it suffers consequences and complications. Female reproductive body skills are not accepted as an item for market exchange. A woman cannot earn money by a surrogacy program. A female body should be subservenient – it should provide help, take care and be altruistic.

Conclusion

This analysis of debates about ARTs in Russia's two most popular newspaper from 1996 to 2006 enables us to assert that a reproductive body is constituted as an overt controlled body of viscera and processes. This effect is achieved as a result of biomedical developments, as Foucault (1998) has shown, and of the developments of medical monitoring technologies (Jonsson 2007; Lauritzen et al. 2007; Rothschild 2006). It is the expansion and spread of monitoring and skin-penetrating technologies that significantly changed attitudes to the body, making it more obvious and extremely controlled (Lauritzen and Hyden 2007: 3).

The language developed in medical practice, as it is communicated in newspapers and in everyday life, allows us to verbalise the body from the inside even when it is impossible to see it. A reproductive body with its reproductive organs, processes and mechanisms is uncovered and made available for monitoring and control not only for professionals, but also for lay readers of printed media. As a result of sight intervention into the body, processes such as conception and pregnancy are desacralised and technologised (Franklin 1998; Lie 2002). Disclosure and description of the reproduction cycle of giving birth to a child makes it possible to normalise ARTs, because they constitute both natural and in vitro fertilisation as symmetric processes. The use of popularised medical and technologised language for body talk creates a common enframing of reproduction.

This leads to autonomy of conception, embryos and fetus, and affirmation of the body as a service-provider for all these processes. As involuntary childlessness is still stigmatised in modern societies – especially for women in Russia's culture of normative motherhood – infertility is perceived as an identity failure (Brednikova and Nartova 2007). Childbirth becomes the primary endpoint. Consequently, fertilisation becomes the main process, with medical and scientific technologies at its service, while a body that is manipulated in many ways to achieve fertilisation is only a resource for a potential child (Rodin and Collins 1991).

In newspaper materials and in practice these discursive tendencies can be easily traced. A reproductive body is not only turned into a service-provider for fertilisation, but also pathologised. The normalisation of ARTs is conducted by means of constituting a dysfunctional reproductive body. This explains why childbirth does not occur unaided any more and why technological interventions are needed. When the reproductive body is reconstituted as an ill body, it requires more control and this legitimises medical power over the whole process of reproduction. The body is subject to more control thorough public monitoring both from the outside and the inside. The female body is most pathologised and this process started several centuries ago (Foucault 1996; Foucault 2002; Michel 2000). This view of the female reproductive body gains power within ART discourse, because it is the female body that is the most manipulated and controlled and that has most responsibility, even though treatments and diagnostics could pursue male infertility or the possible sick condition of the fetus (van Der Ploeg 2004). Thus, reproductive bodies in Russian mass media discourse are produced as dismantled and controlled, dysfunctional bodies. With the help of new reproductive technologies and medical interference, these dysfunctional bodies become resources for achieving conception and childbirth. Ethical, legitimate use of ARTs as a reproductive strategy is limited by two types of unacceptable practices that represent the poles of a continuum of reproductive technology use: cloning and commercialisation.

It is the goal of childbirth that legitimises the use of surrogate motherhood and sperm donation. Affirmation and inclusion of surrogate motherhood and sperm donation into the existing moral and social order is based on the formation of specific body types and body practices involved in these programs. New types of subjectivity are also constituted through the production and normalisation of these specific bodies because, as Foucault (2002) says, a subject is produced through a body by investing power into it.

This analysis shows that both male and female bodies, as well as male and female subjects in surrogate motherhood and sperm donation programs, are produced as almost totally opposite phenomena, even though they are formed within a similar discursive context. Sperm donation leads to male qualification: a donor, a normal and ideal man as confirmed by experts. He sells his body skills and earns money by that, keeping his integrity, protected by anonymity and privacy, and he does not bear the responsibility for the use of his sperm results. Donation infinitely affirms a male subject and a male body.

Surrogate motherhood, to the contrary, leads to disqualification of a female body and a female subject in general. A surrogate body is not only the incorporation of an overt, controlled, public reproductive body, but is also fragmented and defined as a border. It suffers the conflict of interests and aims. Moreover, surrogate motherhood is not represented as a female body skill that can be exchanged for money. Surrogate programs are regulated by the moral code of motherhood: altruism, help, and care (Narayan 1995; Blith and Potter 2003; Ragone 2003). Thus, surrogate motherhood does not celebrate the female body and the female subject, but constitutes it as a perpetual loss and dispersion. It restrains the woman within her earlier reproductive position. At the same time, in the context of sperm donation, male reproduction attains professional status. A donor passes the medical examination, does his job by delivering sperm and is rewarded with money.

The described effects of ART normalisation make the already existing difference in corporeality between men and women even more drastic. Thus it is the male subject that becomes a body, the man is embodied. Masculinity is constituted through an assessment of body quality, through the use of a model of body skills, and through earning money by this model body. The woman appears to be extremely disembodied – she is not perceived within the body, but as a multitude of moral and ethical experiences and categories. Her body qualifications and her body skills are in question, along with her identity, her way of life, her responsibility and her care. Her body is constantly contested and redefined amidst moral debates, plural claims and interests. She is not earning money by her body skills. She helps, saves and serves the children. In media discourse on ARTs, the male body is designated and normalised as a body-property that is subordinate and controlled by the male subject. This is quite in line with the Cartesian differentiation of mind and body, in which the latter is subordinate to former. Contrarily, female bodies are normalised as body-selves (Greil 2002), the space within which the body, the identity and the self are not different and not to be differentiated.

To conclude, I would like to say that the ARTs, including surrogate motherhood, did not bring women either the emancipation or the autonomy that many feminist hoped and fought for (Shanley 1995; Petchesky 1995). The normalisation of ARTs in Russian media discourse only confirms the previously developed 'dispositive' of power, using Michel Foucault's term, with regard to the female body and the female subject, and added some new ones. A female body is still overtly pathologised and controlled. A female subjectivity is still reproduced as altruistic motherhood. Women still do not possess their own bodies and have not escaped forced motherhood. Even in the twenty-first century women are still expected to be an integral unified whole with their body, responsibilities and anxieties, to be an integral self. This might as well become a resource for some of them to achieve inner and external freedom.

References

Blith, E., Potter, C. (2003) Paying for it? Surrogacy, market forces, and assisted conception, in R. Cook, S.D. Sclater and F. Kaganas (eds) *Surrogate Motherhood: International Perspectives.* Oxford, Portland Oregon: Hart Publishing: 227-242.

Brednikova, O. and Nartova, N. (2007) Narushaia molchanie: diskriminatsiia zhenshcnin v prostranstve novyh reproduktivnyh tehnologii (NRT) [Breaking the silence: female discrimination in the realm of new reproductive technologies (NRT)], in O. Zdravomyslova (ed) *Sovremennaia zhenshchina, sem'ia, demographiia: Aktual'nye issledovaniia* [Contemporary Women, Family, Demography: Current Studies]. Moskow: Zven'ia: 156-180.

Cussins, C. (1998) Producing reproduction: techniques of normalisation and naturalization in infertility clinics, in S. Franklin and H. Ragone (eds) *Reproducing Reproduction: Kinship, Power and Technological Innovation*. Philadelphia: University of Pennsylvania Press: 66-101.

Foucault, M. (1996a) Volia k znaniu [The will to fact], in M. Foucault *Volia k istine* [The Will to Truth]. Moskow: Kastal: 97-268.

Foucault M. (1996b) Poraiadok diskursa [The discourse on language], in M. Foucault *Volia k istine* [The Will to Truth]. Moskow: Kastal: 48-95.

Foucault, M. (1998) *Rozhdenie kliniki* [The Birth of the Clinic]. Moscow: Smysl.

Foucault, M. (2002) Vlast' i telo [Pouvoir et corps], in M. Foucault *Intellektualy i vlast': Izbrannye politicheskie stat'i, vystupleniaia i interv'iu* [Intellectuals and Power: Selected Articles, Speeches and Interviews on Politics]. Moskow: Practis: 161-171.

Franklin, S. (1998) Making miracles: scientific progress and facts of life, in S. Franklin and H. Ragone (eds) *Reproducing Reproduction: Kinship, Power and Technological Innovation*. Philadelphia: University of Pennsylvania Press: 102-117.

Greil, A.L. (2002) Infertile bodies: medicalization, metaphor, and agency, in M. C. Inhorn and F. van Balen F. (eds) *Infertility around the Globe: New Thinking on Childlessness, Gender, and Reproductive Technologies*. Berkeley, Los Angeles, London: University of California Press: 101-118.

Jonsson, A. (2007) The normal baby-to-be: lay and professional negotiations of the ultrasound image, in S.O. Lauritzen and L. Hyden (eds) *Medical Technologies and the Life World: The Social Construction of Normality*. London, New York: Routledge, Taylor and Francis Group: 93-114.

Landau, R. and Blyth, E. (1988) Summary and conclusions, in R. Landau R. and E. Blyth (eds) *Third Party Assisted Conception Across Cultures: Social, Legal and Ethical perspectives*. London and New York: Jessica Kindley Publishers: 266-276.

Lauritzen, S.O. and Hyden, L. (2007) Medical technologies, the life world and normality: an introduction, in S.O. Lauritzen and L. Hyden (eds) *Medical Technologies and the Life World: The Social Construction of Normality*. London, New York: Routledge, Taylor and Francis Group: 1-17.

Lauritzen, S.O., Ohman, S.G., Saltvedt, S. A normal pregnancy? Women's experiences of being at high risk after ultrasound screening for Down syndrome, in S.O. Lauritzen and L. Hyden (eds) *Medical Technologies and the Life World: The Social Construction of Normality*. London, New York: Routledge, Taylor and Francis Group: 115-140.

Lie, M. (2002) Science as father? Sex and gender in the age of reproductive technologies, *The European Journal of Women's Studies*, 9(4): 381-399.

Michel, D. (2000) *Voploschennyi chelovek: zapadnaia cultura, medicinskii kontrol' i telo* [The Embodied Human Being: Western Culture, Medical Control and the Body]. Saratov: Izdatel'stvo Saratovskogo Universiteta.

Narayan, U. (1995) The 'gift' of a child: commercial surrogacy, gift surrogacy, and motherhood, in P. Boling (ed) *Expecting Trouble: Surrogacy, Fetal Abuse and New Reproductive Technologies*. Boulder, San Francisco, Oxford: Westview Press: 177-202.

Petchesky, R.P. (1995) The body as property: a feminist re-vision, in F.D. Ginsburg and R. Rapp (eds) *Conceiving the New World Order: The Global Politics of Reproduction*. Berkeley, Los Angeles, London: University of California Press: 387-406.

Ragone, H. (2003) The gift of life: surrogate motherhood, gamete donation and construction of altruism, in R. Cook, S.D. Sclater and F. Kaganas (eds) *Surrogate Motherhood: International Perspectives*. Oxford, Portland Oregon: Hart Publishing: 209-226.

Rodin, J. and Collins, A. (1991) The new reproductive technologies: overview of challenges and issues, in J. Rodin and A. Collins (eds) *Women and New Reproductive Technologies: Medical, Psychosocial, Legal and Ethical Dilemmas*. Hillsdale, New Jersey, Hove and London: Lawrence Erlbaum Associate Publishers: 1-10.

Rothschild, J. (2006) Prenatal diagnosis and disability: the ultimate 'technological fix'? in A. Bamme, G. Getzinger and B. Wieser (eds) *Yearbook 2006 of the Institute for Advanced Studies on Science, Technology and Society*. Graz, München, Wien: Profil: 217-244.

Shanley, M.L. (1995) 'Surrogate mothering' and women's freedom: a critique of contracts for human reproduction, in P. Boling (ed.) *Expecting Trouble: Surrogacy, Fetal Abuse and New Reproductive Technologies*. Boulder, San Francisco, Oxford: Westview Press: 156-176.

van der Ploeg, I. (2004) 'Only angels can do without skin': on reproductive technology's hybrids and the politics of body boundaries, *Body & Society*, 10(2-3): 153-181.

Zdravomyslova, E. and Temkina, A. (2002) Analiz narrativa: vozmozhnosti rekonstrukcii seksual'noi identichnosti [Narrative analysis: the possibilities of sexual identity reconstruction], in E. Zdravomyslova and A. Temkina (eds) *V poiskah seksual'nosti* [In Search of Sexuality]. St. Petersburg: Dmirty Bulanin: 549-558.

In vitro fertilisation in Switzerland: gendered normalisation practices

Andrea Früh

> Well, it gets, it becomes normality, it becomes more normal.
> Manuela, mother of two children after IVF

The ideal of having a family – or rather a nuclear family consisting of a married heterosexual couple with two to three children – is common in Swiss culture. At the same time, the number of children in Swiss families is decreasing[1] and since the 1990s a variety of family patterns can be found (Hoffmann-Nowotny and Höpflinger 1996: 620). As a result of this contradictory situation, a public debate on infertility, demographics and family structures has evolved. In a society where the demographics of the decreasing population are highly debated and the value of the nuclear family in father-mother-child form remains high, childlessness can easily become a stigma, especially for women. It is socially tolerated for men to follow their professional career without having a family or without having children, whereas women, especially married women or women in a partnership, are expected to be mothers. The female biography is perceived as incomplete if it lacks motherhood. In the case of unwanted childlessness, this stigma is especially hard to bear for many women.

Assisted reproductive technologies (ARTs) are a controversial, but appealing, way to overcome unwanted childlessness. The high emotional value of children and the social pressure on couples to reproduce has allowed ARTs – and in the Swiss context especially in vitro fertilisation (IVF) – to become a profitable business. In Switzerland, IVF has been practiced for much more than 20 years, and it is the most prevalent technique, besides the more sophisticated intracytoplasmic sperm injection (ICSI), where a single sperm is chosen and directly injected into an ovum. Every year, between 900 and 1,400 babies are born after IVF and ICSI in Switzerland.[2] Nevertheless, assisted reproduction is still not publicly accepted as a strategy to become a parent. Compared to other European countries such as Spain or Great Britain, and certainly compared to the United States, where this market is not regulated by law, Swiss laws on ARTs are restrictive (see also chapter on ARTs in Switzerland).

The desire to have a child and the handling of infertility are personal issues and at the same time irrevocably bound up with public attitudes towards fertility, conception, and family (Krones 2005: 26ff.). Because the use of ARTs is not yet perceived as just a normal way of conception, women who use ARTs challenge personal and public social norms. Empirical evidence shows that the diagnosed infertility and later the decision to use ARTs are experienced as ruptures in their biography by the women concerned (Früh 2006). Ruptures in this context means deviations from individual or public norms that underlie the personal ideas of 'the normal female biography'.

This article takes the empirical data of biographical interviews with Swiss women who have become mothers after IVF or ICSI (2006)[3] and examines the strategies of these women in integrating the deviating circumstances of their conception – the ruptures – into their biography. Charis Thompson (formerly Cussins), calls these strategies of legitimisation in the case of ARTs 'normalisation' (Cussins 1998; Thompson 2005). Analysis of ruptures during a *Kinderwunschgeschichte*, a wish to have a child and its realisation, and the handling of them, has proven to be a fruitful way of exploring different normalisation strategies used by the women in the present sample.

Assisted reproductive technologies are indisputably a form of high-end medicine. Conception without sexual intercourse has become possible and gives consumers the opportunity to challenge, and maybe even redevelop, social norms. But the concepts of conception and family are loaded with moral principles. Therefore the following analyses will try to prove that it is not the newness and innovation of ARTs in general that are normalised by the women, but rather that normalisation techniques allow the reinterpretation of formerly deviant technical procedures as 'as good as normal', and are rendered socially accepted. This would mean that changes in social practices are not necessarily followed by changes in individual or wider social norms.

The first section of this article gives some more information about normalisation strategies in the context of IVF based on the concepts identified by Thompson (2005), explaining how new technologies and other deviations from the common concept of a *Kinderwunschgeschichte* can be reinterpreted to fit normative expectations. Then, the most prevalent normalisation strategies which were put into practice by the women in the present sample are discussed in detail: reproduction of the nuclear family and naturalisation as strategies of normalisation; naturalisation through the orientation on norms within the clinical setting of ARTs and amongst the patients; and normalisation through the reproduction of gender stereotypes.

About the concept of normalisation

Assisted reproductive technologies have the potential to overthrow the existing paradigm of conception and family relations. They offer a wide field of possible ways to conceive and to become a parent. Fertilisation of the ovum in a test tube makes it possible to choose which sperm and ovum shall be used to create an embryo, as well as which embryo, and how many of them, will be implanted. Biological and social parenthood can thus be divided between different individuals and no longer depend on sexual intercourse between a man and a woman. Singles as well as homosexuals have now the option to become a parent. However, as mentioned above, Swiss law prohibits the use of ARTs to their full potential[4]. Ovum donation and surrogacy are illegal and therefore motherhood cannot be divided or shared between biological and social parents. The donation of sperm is only legal for married heterosexual couples. Thus, ARTs in the Swiss context only partly challenge given social norms and do not provide true freedom of reproductive choice.

The women interviewed in the present sample perceive ARTs as technologies that enable them to overcome infertility. None of the women intended to use ARTs, in their cases IVF or ICSI,[5] as an act of reproductive choice or as a deliberate breach of social norms. Their family plans corresponded perfectly with the common ideal of the nuclear family. It was diagnosed infertility which sparked the first rupture in their *Kinderwunschgeschichte*. Only after this diagnosis did IVF become relevant for them. The use of ARTs was thereafter perceived as a further rupture of the female biography.

According to Lothar Böhnisch (2002: 200), ruptures in biographies are situations where there is a gap between social expectations and the ability to live up to them. Ruptures are neither abnormal nor harmful, nor do they exclusively appear in the context of ARTs. Böhnisch (2002: 200) highlights that such a crisis is not pathological, but should rather be seen as part of every biography; only ruptures can possibly challenge existing social norms and perhaps trigger social change. In the case of ARTs, every time a rupture appears, women have the choice to either normalise or reinterpret the deviant situation to fit the social norms or interpret it as an alternative to the prevailing norms and accept the deviation as such.

All the women in the sample had to go through a process of adapting their ideal of conception as a sexual act of love between a couple, in order to be able to accept IVF as a legitimate way to realize their wish to have a child and a family. During such a process of normalisation, which is highly individual, many decisions have to be taken. The choices and the decision making processes are influenced by different factors such as social norms; individual norms and ideals; specialist knowledge and advice of gynaecologists and other medical specialists; but also by the individual situation of the women. All the women in the sample managed to develop individual strategies to integrate deviations from the norm with their personal *Kinderwunschgeschichte*. Cussins (1998: 67) describes it as '…the grid of what is already there, and what counts as pre-existing, is produced, recognized, reproduced, and changed over time'.

However, analysis of interviews revealed many different stages of a *Kinderwunschgeschichte*. Normalisation can take place during any of them. It begins at the first stage of family planning, when women abandon contraception, and is completed only when infertility and IVF are successfully normalised. At the time of the interviews some of the women were still in the process of coming to terms with their own story of infertility and IVF even though they were mothers of healthy children. Normalisation probably needs to be seen as a continuum, which is not equally successful in all cases, with different individuals reaching different stages.

Reproduction of the nuclear family as a strategy of normalisation

The data collected from the interviews proved what the international literature has demonstrated before: IVF is not an easy way to conception. Women reported physical and psychological stress, such as pains caused by high doses of hormones and during the operation to implant the fertilised embryo. Waiting periods between different steps of treatment and the pressure of facing low success rates of 23% per treatment cycle[6] caused mental distress. Along with these factors, couples spend large amounts of money on services that are not covered by insurance. At the same time, many women do not consider stopping their treatments until they have realised their ideal family pattern, which in the case of this sample includes two or three children. Claudia explains her own situation:

> Then he [Claudia's husband] talked to me in plain language and asked 'do you really want this [IVF]?', because it is an invasion of the female body. 'Do we want to take that risk?' Well, because there might be side effects and so forth. But I was already at the point, well, I have left those questions aside. To me it was obvious that we will finish what we have already started.

The availability of ARTs in general seems to create an environment where the use of these technologies is embraced rather than questioned (Franklin 1998: 107). It can be very difficult for women to decide against available technologies and to prioritise their own health because those very technologies provide the potential for realising their idealised family patterns. As Thompson (2005: 94) says, many patients of ARTs do not give up before they have tried 'everything'. This applies also to the women in the present sample, though 'everything' does not mean the same for all of the women, and the extent to which the women compromise their own health differs. Susanne, for example, was lucky and fell pregnant immediately after her first cycle of IVF. Sabrina, on the other hand, went through a range of treatments for eight years while trying to become pregnant. Both of the women went back for other IVF treatments after the birth of their first child, because they wanted a family with two or three children.

The individual limits of what treatments and side effects are acceptable are arranged on a continuum and shift during the treatment, depending on advice from infertility specialists; personal notions of conception; and on the success of the treatments. Manuela, a biologist and mother of two children, reflected on her own process during IVF. She was convinced that no woman can foresee how much pain and psychological pressure she would endure to realise her *Kinderwunsch* in case of infertility. From her own experience, she knows that ideals can be adapted to the real situation and the urge to live the desired family life can be very powerful. The decision to use IVF is not the result of a single, conscious decision, but rather that of an ongoing normalisation process. Sometimes personal ideals prove hard to abandon; but as we will see in the next section, individuals can be very creative in normalising the 'abnormal'.

Naturalisation as a strategy of normalisation

The *Kinderwunsch* suggests a 'natural' desire, independent from any cultural dispositions or social influences (Hauser-Schäublin 2001: 207). It is perceived as an anthropological component of human life. Assisted reproductive technologies, as a technological way to have a child, disturb this image and therefore need to be naturalised in order to be normalised and accepted. A society that looks at conception as something deeply natural must naturalise the treatments connected with fertility and infertility to preserve the ideal of conception as a deeply natural event. Thompson (2005: 141) describes this process of naturalisation thus:

> Reading new ways of getting pregnant and starting families onto a conventional model of the normative (in this country nuclear) family is a strategy that is commonly used to achieve this [normalisation].

Different strategies are available to naturalise IVF. However, one basic strategy was used by all women in the sample to naturalise this highly technical treatment. What used to be promoted as a technical revolution in medicine, namely to impregnate the ovum with the sperm outside the female body – in vitro as the name says – was reinterpreted. The focus was moved from the striking fact that IVF takes place outside the female body. Rather, the women emphasised that everything else during an IVF impregnation is exactly the same as during any other conception. Therefore, they argue that IVF is as good as natural, and thus normal. In the case of ICSI, where the sperm that impregnates the ovum is selected by a specialist, this naturalisation process proves to be more difficult as the example of Manuela and her husband shows:

> And then he [her husband] did not think it was good for me [IVF]. He looked at it as too unnatural. An insemination means that you have your own menstrual cycle which you support with hormones, but only very little. Well, and your insurance pays for it three times, and it's really still more or less – normal (laughing softly). And the other option [IVF] is relatively unna[tural] – well, it's all controlled.

Manuela and her husband, both trained biologists, made the factor of naturalness the key factor for their decisions which ART treatments they would use to realise their *Kinderwunsch*. However, the fact that insemination appeared to them as more natural than IVF did not mean that the procedure could not be normalised at all. After much research in scientific journals and many discussions, Manuela's husband agreed to IVF treatments. Yet he was still not prepared to agree on ICSI, because he viewed the human selection of the sperm to impregnate an ovum as an excessive interference with nature, which would be unhealthy also. Manuela and her husband agreed on this compromise.

Other couples normalised ICSI, arguing that the development of the embryo, and later the fetus, happens without human influence, thus naturally. Naturalisation is a question of interpretation. From a statistically perspective, it is true that ICSI bears more risks for the fetus than IVF. Thus many women prefer to use IVF without ICSI. But again, different ARTs can be placed on a continuum. As Thompson (2005: 141) puts it: '(...) patients go through their own changes over time about what seems natural and acceptable and what seems frighteningly or impossibly unnatural.' The following examples show how individual naturalisation can take place and how concepts of nature can shift over time.

Sabrina first defined IVF as unnatural and wrong from a religious point of view. After she learnt about her husband's infertility and failed to fall pregnant despite several inseminations, Sabrina was still not prepared to use IVF. She argued that God would have helped her to conceive naturally if he wanted her to have a child. Thus she explained her childlessness and her unsuccessful efforts as the will of a higher, divine power. But two years later, after collecting a great deal of information about IVF, Sabrina managed to normalise the procedure. She legitimised IVF by saying that God would not have allowed the scientists to develop this technology if it was unnatural or wrong. Not only the moral side of IVF, but also the initially mentioned lack of naturalness, was normalised that way.

In Susanne's case the naturalisation process only set in when she gave birth. Susanne very much wanted to give birth 'naturally', without technical interventions such as a Caesarean section. Giving birth to her child naturally was her way to naturalise IVF and the connected treatments. Susanne depended very much on using this normalisation strategy. However, because of complications during labour, she needed an emergency Caesarean and thus failed to give birth 'naturally'. This rupture in her plans caused a profound crisis that other women have experienced at earlier stages of the treatment and forced Susanne to actively start normalisation in different ways.

Normalisation within the norms of the clinic and among patients

Not only the patients but also their suppliers, the numerous fertility specialists and fertility clinics as well as the pharmaceutical companies that sell the drugs for the treatments, promote IVF as a 'close to natural' treatment. Nevertheless, these technologies are relatively new and neither fertility specialists nor patients know much about side effects, and even less about long-term effects. Everybody reacts differently to the numerous drugs and therapies, and psychological factors interfere as well. Women cannot make their decisions for or against certain treatments by relying on common social norms, because IVF deviates from those norms. Thus they often compare themselves with other IVF patients and rely on standards which are defined within the setting of the clinic. Patients as well as physicians define the norms within the fertility clinic and look for new parameters to guide their decision making. Thus, normalisation within the standards of the clinic reassures the women that they are doing the right thing. An exceptionally powerful tool for this normalisation is statistical data, which offers an objective picture of a complex situation. In moments of desperation and failure, women find strength and new hope in those figures and probabilities. Manuela, for example, looked at the situation from a statistical point of view, after her first IVF treatment did not lead to a pregnancy:

> We knew we could try again later. And we knew that the chances for success are only twenty percent the first time.

Manuela focussed on the twenty percent chances of success and judged the first failure as normal. Not only quantitative information, but also the emphasis on certain quality standards empowered the women to continue their treatments, and let them judge their situation within the broader picture of IVF outcomes. Sabrina's statement shows how much weight is put on those indicators and also how powerful the analyses and predications of fertility specialists are:

> And he [Sabrina's fertility specialist] told me I had wonderful follicles. Thus I thought that surely they have all been fertilised well. Even now I don't know why they did not last.

Even specialist knowledge cannot always provide reliable estimations of the situation, but they still normalise the women's performance in terms of statistical norms and level of performance within the setting of ARTs.

Not only statistical information about IVF and measurable quality standards, but the comparison of their own situation with the situation of other women experiencing infertility and IVF treatments helps the women in dealing with their *Kinderwunschgeschichte*. To have a peer group that shares norms, even if they deviate from the common social norms, makes it easier to apply normalisation processes and accept IVF. However, within the realm of ARTs there are treatments that are more, and others that are less, easily normalised by the patients. The most evident example, as discussed before, is uncertainty about ICSI, which is a widespread technology even though statistics show that the risks for abnormalities are higher compared to simpler treatments.

Norms within IVF are not only set by statistics, but also by normative expectations of who is a legitimate mother. One factor is the age of the women at which they decide to do IVF. Sally, for example, felt that her wish to use IVF was not taken seriously by fertility specialists because she was only 23 years old at her first attempt, even though she had previously undergone infertility treatments and her partner was diagnosed infertile. Sally was advised to be patient because from the perspective of the infertility specialists, she still had many years left to try. Because of her young age, Sally did not fit into the narrow frame of the 'normal' IVF patient. She had to legitimate her right to use ARTs before she was accepted as a patient. Susanne experienced the same problem but at the opposite end of age limitations. After she had given birth to two children through IVF, she wanted to have a third treatment four years later, when she was 42. She was told that the chances of an IVF pregnancy are very low after the age of 40. Even though she had conceived immediately at the age of 37 and 38, her specialist only agreed to provide one more IVF cycle and refused any further treatment afterwards. Those examples show that there are normative expectations concerning the age of the patients which are regarded as pivotal parameters for defining the boundaries of legitimate IVF treatments by physicians. Thus, the normalisation of IVF, as well as the access to it, is not only a question of availability, even within the legal guidelines, but also depends on the individual parameters such as the assessment of physicians which cannot be influenced by the women.

Normalisation through the reproduction of gender stereotypes

Gender roles in Swiss culture during the 1990s were defined more traditionally after the birth of the first child than in childless relationships (Hoffmann-Nowotny and Höpflinger 1996: 614). In the case of the present study, this tendency is evident as well, even though these women had very different biographies. All of them were prepared to step back from their jobs and put their time and energy into being a mother, at least for some time. The anthropological component of motherhood as a natural female role was not questioned after the use of highly technological treatments such as IVF. The reproduction of the stereotypical female role of being a mother was rather welcomed by the women as a normalisation strategy. Susanne, for example, was determined to part with her successful professional career after the birth of her first child:

> I am not a person who says, I want a child, to continue working fulltime, using daycares and nannies and everything. Under such circumstances I don't need a child.

Generally it can be said that the women interviewed felt very much obliged to be 'good' mothers and to make their children's wellbeing their first priority. As Claudia's example shows, she felt privileged to have a child after IVF and saw it as her motherly duty to take on this role without complaining:

> Such situations as colic [in the baby] are surely easier to accept after having experienced an assisted reproduction. Because one knows what price the whole thing had. And you tell yourself that it is not self-evident that you have a child in your arms that you need to carry around and to comfort somehow. It has another significance, I think.

Claudia fully identified with the role of the competent and caring mother. Even though social norms have changed over time and have become more flexible, Sabrina's story shows how narrow the boundary between the socially desired and the intolerable can be. Sabrina gave up her professional work during the exhausting ARTs. Her physician recommended that she reduce stress, as it decrees the possibility of pregnancy. Although Swiss society places a certain value on a woman who does not continue her professional career once she is a mother, women who have neither a job nor a child to look after do not fit into the social norm. Sabrina explained her situation as follows:

> I felt stupid. Really, I felt I needed to legitimate to the public that I did not work, and I did not have a child or anything. What did I do the whole day? Sit at home.

Normalising motherhood means fitting into a picture of the female role model in general, even before a child is born.

Women who use IVF are very much aware of the social norms that define a stereotypical female biography: the importance of being a mother and the duty to be a good mother. The reproduction of gender stereotypes is used as a strategy to normalise IVF, in other words to avoid more deviations, and normalisation work after the conception through IVF. But to assume that this division of roles is static would be wrong. The interviews showed that it can be a temporary strategy, as in the case of Manuela, who went back to work after the birth of her first child, or Claudia, who started giving courses for baby massages when she was a mother. Those examples show that ruptures in biography are not only defined by the public, but can also be defined and redefined on a personal level.

Conclusions and perspectives

The interviewed women proved that the human ability to integrate deviant situations during a *Kinderwunschgeschichte* where ARTs are used is high. These women have developed various ways of normalising ARTs within their personal biography, and have succeeded in reinterpreting deviant elements. Instead of promoting IVF as a new way of conception, women found their own ways of normalising IVF without challenging existing concepts of conception, fertility and family. Thus, the interviewed women did not deviate from the concept of nuclear family and they even reproduced the apparent return towards stereotypical gender roles generally observed in couples after the birth of their first child – at least for a limited amount of time. Furthermore, they normalised IVF by naturalising so-called 'artificial reproduction'. They reinterpreted fertilisation outside the body as a close-to-natural way of procreation with the argument that actual impregnation of the ovum takes place exactly the same way as inside the body, with the only difference that this happens in the test tube. However, ICSI failed to be normalised by the women to the same extent as simpler IVF treatments. They perceived ICSI as 'less natural than IVF' because the sperm that impregnated the ovum is chosen by humans, and also internalised statistical evidence that indicates the procedure is more dangerous for the health of the fetus. The latter shows that the development of new technologies and treatments will provide patients and fertility experts with challenges in normalising innovative procedures.

As the analysis has shown, normalisation processes often reproduce shared social norms such as the nuclear family, and rather stereotypical gender roles. But it must be stressed that normalisation strategies do vary accordingly to personal factors such as age, social background or social environment, and that norms are not static, but change according to these personal factors. The women were very flexible in working out rationales and explanations for their actions or decisions, and every time their situation changes the reasoning needs to be adapted.

During treatment, there were two settings where the female IVS patients experienced norms differing from the prevailing public social expectations that supported them in their normalisation process. The first setting was the fertility clinic, and the fertility treatments in general; during those treatments the women and the specialists referred to norms that emerged out of the setting of the infertility treatment. Statistical knowledge especially was used to set new standards and thus normalise IVF within the setting of the clinic. The infertility specialists provided further assistance through normalisation processes, but also put into place normative rules within the ARTs. The second setting was the in-group consisting of other women who have used IVF to become mothers and of the infertility specialists. Whether those women met on the internet forums or personally, they did not need to start normalising IVF from the scratch. They referred to the norms within IVF to help manage their sense of deviance.

Social norms in general are not static; but outsiders have not experienced the whole process of normalisation and are therefore expected to see ARTs as artificial (in terms of normalisation as naturalisation, see Hauser-Schäublin 2001: 97). Not only women using IVF, but also outsiders and the public need to go through processes of normalisation. If ARTs can be accepted as a new way of conception by users and by the society, there will not be a need anymore to use normalisation strategies in order to integrate ARTs within female biographies. But as Faye Ginsberg and Rayna Rapp (1995: 10) have explained, social transformations are not self-evident because human beings often do not want changes in their lives.

Generally, scholarly work and public debate on infertility and ARTs mostly focus on female patients. It would be interesting to conduct further research into gendered perspectives of IVF and infertility in general. Assisted reproductive technologies as well as fertility in general are highly gendered areas and it would be interesting to gain more insight into male perspectives on fertility and related treatments. The women of this sample were lucky to fall pregnant after IVF, considering the rather low success rates; but infertility and the ensuing ART procedures were still considered a major rupture within their individual biographies, and the normalisation processes took much longer than the actual medical treatments. Not only IVF has to be normalised, but also infertility itself and the fact that life courses can only be planned to a certain extent. We need discussions about infertility, not only about ARTs, before the latter can become accepted.

Further research is also needed on the long-term development of gender roles after the birth of a child and on normalisation processes in the longer term. It is quite possible that gender roles will be assigned differently again after the children have grown up – and this includes couples that have not used ARTs. As the 'facts of life' in the case of IVF deviate from what is commonly understood by the term, naturalisation as normalisation might again emerge as a topic when children who were born after IVF want to know about their own origin.

Notes

[1] Bundesamt für Statistik, Indikatoren der Fruchtbarkeit in der Schweiz, (su-d-01.02.02.03.01.01), http://www.bfs.admin.ch/bfs/portal/de/index/themen/01/06/blank/data/01.html (last accessed November 17, 2006).

[2] Bundesamt für Statistik (ed.). 2006. Statistik der medizinisch unterstützten Fortpflanzung. Neuchâtel, http://www.bfs.admin.ch/bfs/portal/de/index/news/publikationen.html?publicationID=2433 (last accessed November 17, 2006).

[3] In 2006, the author conducted qualitative research on the situation of individual ART patients in Switzerland. The main focus was to elaborate on the trajectories of women who conceived after IVF or ICSI from the time when they first planned to have a child up to the day they gave birth. Data was collected during five narrative biographical interviews (Schütze 1983) with five women. These interviews were analysed in-depth with Bohnsack's (2000) documentary method. The aim was to define different stages during a history of overcoming childlessness as well as to investigate personal decision-making processes and the normalisation processes which had taken place. Referring to Thompson (2005: 92) infertility was not reduced to a 'major life crisis', as is often done by psychologists, but emphasis was placed on fertility as a rupture in biography that questions the idealised female biography. All interviewees live in the German-speaking part of Switzerland and were married by the time of the interview.

They were between 23 and 36 years old when they began treatment. Some women were very involved in a professional career, some less. Some of the women had a long history of unwanted childlessness and had made many attempts to overcome infertility with treatments other than ARTs before they chose to turn to IVF or ICSI. In all cases, male factor infertility was the reason for using ARTs. All the women shared the feeling that they did not only want a child, but a family, or a nuclear family. They were prepared to go through several treatment cycles to realise this family model, even though such treatments can be physically and mentally challenging and expensive.

[4] Fortpflanzungsmedizingesetz (FmedG) 1.1.2001

[5] All of the interviewees fell pregnant after IVF. Some of them also used ICSI. When IVF is written, ICSI should be understood to be included. Only in cases where the specific technique of ICSI makes a difference to the argument, is this term used.

[6] Bundesamt für Statistik (ed.). 2006. Statistik der medizinisch unterstützten Fortpflanzung. Neuchâtel. www.bfs.admin.ch/bfs/portal/de/index/news/ publikationen.html?publicationID=2433 (last accessed November 17, 2006).

References

Böhnisch, L. (2002) Lebensbewältigung. Ein sozialpolitisch inspiriertes Paradigma für die Soziale Arbeit, in T. Werner (ed.) *Grundriss Soziale Arbeit: Ein einführendes Handbuch*. Opladen: Leske + Budrich: 199–213.

Bohnsack, R. (2000) *Rekonstruktive Sozialforschung: Einführung in Methodologie und Praxis qualitativer Forschung*. Opladen: Leske + Budrich.

Cussins, C. (1998) Producing reproduction: techniques of normalisation and naturalisation in infertility clinics, in S. Franklin and H. Ragoné (eds) *Reproducing Reproduction: Kinship, Power and Technological Innovation*. Philadelphia: University of Pennsylvania Press: 66–101.

Franklin, S. (1998) Making miracles: scientific progress and the facts of life, in S. Franklin and H. Ragoné (eds) *Reproducing Reproduction: Kinship, Power, and Technological Innovation*. Philadelphia: University of Pennsylvania Press: 102–117.

Früh, A. (2006) *Die Bewältigung des unerfüllten Kinderwunsches bei Frauen im Kontext einer künstlichen Befruchtung: Eine Untersuchung aus sozialpädagogischer Perspektive*. Unpublished MA thesis. Zurich: Pädagogisches Institut.

Ginsburg, F. D., Rapp, R. (1995) Introduction: conceiving the new world order, in F. D. Ginsburg and R. Rapp (eds) *Conceiving the New World Order: The Global Politics of Reproduction*. Berkeley: University of California Press: 1–17.

Hauser-Schäublin, B. (2001) *Der geteilte Leib: Die kulturelle Dimension von Organtransplantation und Reproduktionsmedizin in Deutschland.* Frankfurt/New York: Campus Verlag.

Hoffmann-Nowotny, H.-J., Höpflinger, F. (1996) Status of family theory and research in Switzerland', in M. B. Sussman and R.S. Hanks (eds), *Intercultural Variation in Family Research and Theory: Implications for Cross-National Studies,* Vol. II. New York, London: Haworth Press: 599–626.

Schütze, F. (1983) Biographieforschung und narratives Interview, *Neue Praxis.* 13: 283–293.

Thompson, Ch. (2005) *Making Parents: The Ontological Choreography of Reproductive Technologies.* London: Cambridge Press.

Reproductive technologies, parenthood and families

Finally parents: normalising infertility and reproductive treatment in Switzerland

Zora Schaad

> Technologies derive from and are created by cultural priorities. Parenthood is one such priority. It is easy to see why new reproductive technologies have caught on so quickly: they hold the potential to allow people to reproduce themselves by having a child.
> Gay Becker, *The Elusive Embryo: How women and men approach new reproductive technologies,* 2000: 11

Many couples try to fulfil their dream of a family with the aid of assisted reproductive technologies (ARTs). Infertility or unwanted childlessness disturbs life plans and is regarded as a rupture in one's biography and gender identity (Ginsburg and Rapp 1995; Becker 2000; Thompson 2005). Assisted reproduction is sought as a means to regain normality. This article aims to trace the normalisation and naturalisation strategies of unwanted childless couples in Switzerland. In this study I detected strategies of normalisation before, during and after treatment (see also Schaad 2008). They are used, amongst other strategies, with the intention of constituting infertility as a widespread, rather than self-inflicted, phenomenon and as a means of achieving conformity to an idealised picture of a 'normal' family and normative biography. In this chapter three kinds of normalisation and naturalisation of infertility and ARTs are presented: biographical normalisation; social normalisation; and normalisation with the goal of embedding circumstances of infertility and ART treatment in a wider context.

Interviews were conducted with six Swiss couples just after they had become parents by using ARTs. Access to these couples was gained through the assistance of a midwife. Interviews focused on themes related to ARTs, infertility, and the wish for a child. Generally, the women were more willing to talk about infertility and ARTs than the men (Hadolt 2003). Informants were between thirty-five and forty-nine years old, thus above the average of twenty-nine years for primiparous women in Switzerland (BFS 2006: 6). All informants were middle or upper class. Their periods of involuntarily childlessness lasted between three and twelve years. The couples' chosen treatments were homologous insemination, hormonal stimulation and intracytoplasmic sperm injection (ICSI). All the babies were delivered by Caesarean section. Six of the twelve persons wished to have one or two other children, three were still undecided, and two did not specify.

Normalisation as an analytic tool

According to Charis Thompson (2005: 80) the concept of normalisation incorporates the ideas of what is 'normal', 'normative' and 'natural'. Things are considered normal when they are present in a condition in which we are accustomed to seeing them. Norms are institutional and moral prescriptions that justify and direct social behaviour, specifically, the actions of infertility patients in this case. Contemporary experiences of infertility as much as reproductive treatments themselves

> are conceptualized and structured around a strongly coupled, heterosexual, consumer-oriented, normative nuclear-family scenography. When successful, treatment enables women [and couples] to reinscribe themselves into that logic. (Thompson 2005: 55).

Norms are usually based upon some degree of consensus, and a failure to conform to widely accepted norms can cause social sanctions. The concept of normalisation describes processes in which new social data, such as new patients, knowledge and instruments, are incorporated into pre-existing procedures; but also includes the ways in which these data are produced, recognised, reproduced, and changed (2005: 80). According to this model, naturalisation can be understood as

> the rendering of states of affairs and facts in a scientific or biological idiom and to the means by which aspects of the site are rendered unproblematic or self-evident in the sense of seeming 'natural'. (Thompson 2005: 80-81)

Physicians control the normality of a patient's body with the aid of appropriate 'topographic knowledge', which is embodied in skilled gestures, the alignment of instruments and the use of specific terminology (Thompson 2005: 81, 193). As long as normality is given or can be re-established, patients are classified as capable of treatment and for a future pregnancy.

Thompson (2005: 71) states that infertility patients often display exaggerated stereotypical gender attributes 'perhaps to signal their fitness to become heterosexual nuclear parents and probably also to rescue gender and sexual identities.' The decision – made by politics, medical specialists, and public opinion – as to whether a couple is suitable for treatment and parenting is based on the supposed well-being of the child to be 'created'. However, the performance of traditional gender specific roles is expected within medical sites. Men for example, whose part is generally reduced to an 'ejaculatory role', were demanded to show compliance, by accompanying their partner, for example (Thompson 2005: 121, 133).

Normalisation processes also occur with respect to the attitudes of the persons involved. In vitro fertilisation (IVF), for example, came to seem very normal and natural. As a result of higher success rates, many babies were born with the assistance of this technology, and more complex ARTs such as intracytoplasmic sperm injection (ICSI) were developed. Awareness of the difficulties that can emerge during the process of conception is closely related to the character of the reproductive treatment during which the infertile body is constantly observed, analysed and qualified.

The tentativeness of both 'normal' and assisted reproduction and the continuing expansion of reproductive medicine transforms the application of ARTs increasingly to the 'normal' case of conception (Franklin 1998: 104-106). Thompson (2005: 141) states that 'a successful way to make new things seem normal is to interpret them as new examples of old things.' This process '(…) normalizes and domesticates procedures, making them seem like appropriate ways of building a family rather than monstrous innovations.' My analysis will show that infertility is often experienced as a failure to perform gendered roles and as an obstacle to a 'normal' life. Women experience infertility as a profound role malfunction and tend to be interested in overcoming infertility, while their husbands focus on returning to normalcy, either by pursuing or ceasing treatment. These gendered patterns appear regardless of which partner had the reproductive impairment, as is also shown in the literature (Greil 1988: 192). The application of ARTs can – if successful – reestablish 'normality' but is often kept secret since it does not represent the putatively ideal and normal way of starting a family.

Biographical normalisation

The term 'biographical normalisation' encompasses actions and statements that constitute attempts to adjust to gender and class specific 'normal biographies', a concept that can be traced back to Levy (1977). Normal biographies include patterns of standardised life courses that have emerged in contemporary times and are characterised by institutionalised sequences of biographical, gendered steps. The chronological order is generally divided into education, work, and retirement. For women, an orientation towards the female normal biography can be detected in references to employment interruption when a child is born (Levy 1977: 44; Hager 2006: 24). In Euro-American societies, family and marriage – which is usually considered as prerequisite for the later birth of children, an understanding echoed by many of my interviewees – is given high priority in life plans.

> Enzo. It became clear to me that Janine was the right one and yes, in this case, also for having children. I only married because of children.

The connection between marriage and starting a family is an intrinsic feature of Levy's (1977) normal biography, which describes family as consisting of a woman and a man, generally married, with shared biological children and domicile. Although ARTs allow new combinations of familial arrangements with specific implications for the social life of the affected individuals and society, my informants strive to achieve the normative, traditional family form. Regardless of adherence to these old forms and ideas – which I regard as normalisation and traditionalism – ARTs encompass the potential for unsettling pictures we have previously taken for granted.

> In so far as the NRTs enable Euro-Americans to do things they could never have done before, they bring new sets of assumptions into place, and in doing so create the sense of conservatism that is attached to the old. (…) In so far as the NRT's [sic] intervene the processes of procreation, then, they do not simply validate old representations of what kinship is about. They have the potential to make us think again about what we take for granted, what we look for in family life, how we regard the relationship between parents and children. (Strathern 1999: 180)

The persistence of traditional patterns must not necessarily be interpreted as conservatism, but can also be understood as a means of reinterpreting old forms (Thompson 2005); and thus a process that helps embed potentially frightening innovations into comfortable world views. I use the notion of embedding, re-embedding and dis-embedding according to Giddens (1991). His concept is well-known in various social science disciplines and refers to a process whereby social relationships are removed from local contexts of interaction and restructured 'across indefinite spans of time-space' (Giddens 1991: 21). Introducing changed practices and life situations into accustomed settings requires its practical embedding in structures and working practices and its enculturing in shared norms and values.

The above mentioned preference of biological parenthood is part of a set of norms around reproduction and is also reflected by legislation (Johnson 1999: 47; Becker 2000: 65; FmedG 2006). The aim of genetic relation represents something Alessandra wanted to achieve.

> Alessandra: I wanted to marry someday and have children. (…) When I found Mr. Right I wanted something that consisted of him and me, a small creature that maybe had the same traits as me or papa's character.

Consanguine kin is still considered primordial. Assisted reproduction technologies exert pressure on the dominant kinship system that distinguishes between appropriate and inappropriate relatives through naturalisation (Knecht 2003: 53). At the same time, ARTs provide the opportunity to stick to the criterion of biological offspring and thereby subordinate other forms of solidarity. My informants judge adoption as the only a 'second best' option (Onnen-Isemann 2000). Cyril, for example, imagines adopting a child after the birth of his first biological daughter. Even in outlining the contours of a possible adoptive child, Cyril pursues strategies of normalisation and naturalisation.

> Cyril: My wife hoped for a girl, I didn't care. I'd prefer to have a child where you can't see at first glance that it isn't our child, if possible. That only makes things worse. It [the child] already bears the burden of being adopted and being of black or Asian descent complicates things further… for integration in school and everywhere. (…) I'd prefer a European child – the younger, the better.

Adoption is only considered when all other options for a biological child have been exhausted. In a fashion similar to that of biological offspring, it is hoped that the adopted child will enter into the family at as young an age as possible and will share physical attributes with his or her new parents. Cyril's position might be based on a fear that he would not be able to adequately apply normalising strategies and fully accept a child that does not fulfil his desired criteria. To sum up, the choice of ARTs did not induce interviewees to abandon ideals that belong to the culturally hegemonic normal biography and its norms concerning parenthood. Establishing a stable relationship between two heterosexual partners – usually married – is reckoned the preliminary stage on the imagined life course before starting a family.

Application of ARTs to advance on an imagined life trajectory is also associated with ideas of nature.

> On the one hand, men and women were prepared to accept (...) that technology could be used to 'improve' on biology/nature. On the other hand, the couples could conceive of these improvements as acceptable so long as the changes to 'nature' were true to its principles. In other words, one could 'give

> nature a helping hand', as in the case of people having difficulty conceiving children, but this help should go to heterosexual couples: the 'natural' context for conceiving children. (Hirsch 1999: 92).

The notion of the family includes kinship relations that are based on shared substances and a duogenetic model of reproduction. My informants did not exclude adoption as a last resort, though they made efforts to try everything to create biological offspring and a natural family. Whether the persistence of these norms is connected to the comparatively restrictive system of reproductive treatment in Switzerland – it is limited to heterosexual, putatively stable, young, solvent couples – or an expression of our society's general condition, cannot be judged on the basis of my sample. Non-hegemonic forms of postmodern kinship – 'patchwork' families, children with homosexual parents or those who were created with the aid of egg donation, etc. – are present in our midst, but do not form an apparent patient group in local infertility clinics. Quite visible, however, is the group to which my informants belong, which does not show great deviation from widespread collective biographies, but rather considerable adherence to an ideology of the technological feasibility of a longed-for child.

Still, I think that normalisation strategies not only hearken back to a conservative pattern of maintaining old beliefs, but should also be regarded against the background of unwanted childlessness and the successful application of these strategies. This suggests, in my view, a new calmness in dealing with reproduction and ARTs. After all, these technologies lead to an avoidance of sexual intercourse which, according to Strathern (2001: 363), is seen as an important element for the establishment of kinship and intimacy. It is noteworthy, however, that my informants did not experience any form of crisis regarding this omission, but reported irrelevance as soon as the pregnancy was achieved. The fact that a family with biological children was the highest ideal while many couples simultaneously considered adoption, shows that naturalisation and socialisation can go together as strategies of establishing kinship (Thompson 2005: 5).

Information management and social normalisation

Strategies of normalisation are often applied with the objective of normalising infertility and ARTs within a given social context. Social normalisation starts with the decision whether to inform anyone, and then who should be told. The importance of information management was stressed repeatedly.

> Sabine: I found it okay to talk to Daniel [husband] and also Daniel said I should not talk about it too much, this is our business. He didn't talk to anybody.

> Linda: Everybody knew about it. My friends more than his friends [referring to her partner Paul]. I frequently talked to my friends about the matter, it came up again and again.

Emotional barriers in communication are found in relation to conception difficulties and the use of ARTs. Women and men report inner resistance and uncertainty about disclosures (Franklin 1997: 122). Most of my informants either did not tell anyone or only partly informed third parties.

> Alessandra: Out of respect for my husband [who had the reproductive impairment] I would not tell anybody. (…) Because if I tell my best friend, she certainly wants to tell to her husband.

> Paul: I don't have problems talking about the matter factually with physicians. But beside this, I did not talk about it much. With my friends, it was somehow disagreeable because it is an intimate theme.

> Carolina: Our friends and acquaintances – I didn't tell them about in vitro and about treatment – disclosure always means questions and uncertainties, and I didn't want to soften on the matter. I just wanted to go through with the thing.

These reasons include a reluctance to talk about intimate subjects; shame; regard for partners; and fears of constant inquiries or insensitive reactions. In all of the cases, discretion was only partial, applied for instance at work, but not to close friends or family. When couples decided to communicate frankly, they generally received good reactions.

> Enzo: I was upfront about it with most people, which was good for me. I didn't have to pretend. My boss at that time was Swiss, but she had lived in Ghana for several years, and then she once went to Africa. I asked whether she could bring an African fertility fetish [laughs]. She then brought along a small figurine but it didn't work because she had already photographed it and thereby desecrated the fetish [laughs]. (…) And when my current boss asked me, he got my standard answer: 'Yes, we do want children but I've reached the limits of my biological capacity [allusion to his sperm quality].' And then it turned out that he had been to the same infertility clinic and is the father of two year old twins now.

Open communication not only provided positive reactions, but also offered opportunities to give accounts of similar cases. After all, dialogue with unaffected people normalises dealing with infertility and ARTs. Discussion helps create and establish new social paths and to reduce a feared stigma. Although my informants were never confronted with direct stigma (Kohler Riessmann 2002: 166), they sometimes experienced insensitive reactions or earned platitudes after disclosure. Several informants reported this kind of reaction and experienced great disappointment, especially regarding their disposition of providing others with confidence. Statements like 'everything is going to be alright' or 'you just need patience, you are too fixed on your wish for a child' shift responsibility upon the infertile. These responses could create anger, given infertile couples' enormous efforts to achieve a pregnancy. On the other hand, my informants knew about the awkwardness trusted third parties might be experiencing, and judged these reactions as attempts at consolation. Such missed efforts can also be seen as the starting point for a deeper conversation, which could support raised awareness and thereby normalise exposure to the matter.

Some of my informants thought that the normalisation of ARTs is merely a matter of time.

> Alessandra: The notion of the artificial insemination is quite common. If you had one, then you are like… artificial! And this is even stronger in the older generation.

In this opinion, Alessandra is in agreement with Becker (2000: 19):

> Today babies such as Louise Brown are seen as a normal part of life. People have adjusted to the idea that conception may take place in the lab, not in the womb. In twenty years new reproductive technologies have not only come full circle, they have come to be viewed around the world as simply another means of conception.

Although increasing use of ARTs will probably eventually lead to normalisation, Alessandra does not intend to tell her daughter about how she was conceived. However, the majority of my interviewees planned to inform their child and were sure that this revelation would not attract interest in the future.

> Linda: I visited the children in school [where she teaches] together with Moritz [her baby]. And then, a first-grader asked how I gave birth. I said I'd had a Caesarean and then many children said [imitates children's voices] 'I am a Caesarean, too; I am also a Caesarean!' It was so cute! I think these children were told frankly about their birth and I think that this will also happen here [referring to ARTs].

Linda's speculations are strengthened by the increasing number of women treated with ARTs in Switzerland (BFS 2006: 8; Hohl 2003: 328), and by active research in different disciplines along with media attention given to the topic. There is a need to find social forms to deal with the subject because of the increasingly prominent cultural and social meanings of ARTs in Switzerland and elsewhere. De Jong (2008) overrules the objection that only a minority of persons are affected by the outsourcing of reproduction in the lab, referring to Strathern, who stresses that this development provokes a general shift in the thinking about family and kinship, which again implicates public, e.g. legal, consequences. Patients face many reservations concerning disclosure of infertility and use of ARTs. Reproduction and sexuality are viewed as delicate and too intimate to discuss. Reasons for secrecy differ, but they combine anticipations of negative reactions and fears that ARTs might not (yet) be socially accepted.

Contrary to Onnen-Isemann's (2000) data, where most of the women only talked to their husband and gynaecologist about infertility and ART procedures, my interviewees indicate at least one more confidant. I still was surprised by this, considering existing taboos. Given such comparative willingness to communicate in my sample, silence and non-disclosure might be even higher in reality. Sympathetic reactions after disclosure constitute a promising sign towards social normalisation. This development not only suggests a reduction of stigmatisation, but also renders the group of infertile persons more visible and provides them with agency.

Embedding infertility and reproductive treatment

Normalisation strategies are also used to embed circumstances of infertility and ART treatment in a broader context where they do not seem controversial, and to re-establish displaced borders. This levelling is of much importance regarding the life crisis induced by childlessness and reproductive treatment, and also with regard to the still existing taboo of artificial reproduction.

Alessandra for instance distances herself from infertility by emphasising the exogenous reasons for her husband's poor sperm quality.

> Alessandra: I think this is nasty. I mean, maybe you had mumps too late, like my husband – we don't know exactly whether this is the reason [for the low sperm quality] or whether it is due to the chemistry he is exposed to [as haircutter], but I think it is important to support these people. When one can give [nature] a helping hand, I think it's okay.

It is striking that my interviewees frequently locate the 'blame' for infertility outside their responsibilities, for example by stressing their healthy lifestyle. This strategy protects against self-doubt while simultaneously advancing a sense that actors are incapable of changing the situation.

> Interviewer: Before you received the diagnosis of diminished sperm quality; what did you blame for your childlessness?
> Janine: It really was difficult. We don't smoke, we hardly drink. I like a glass of wine sometimes, but really not much. Okay, we don't do much sport and we eat more than enough. But there was nothing we could do. Otherwise you could say, 'stop smoking or drinking,' but we couldn't say that.

Regardless of the diagnosis, each couple had constructed an explanation that left them without blame and responsibility (Kohler Riessmann 2002: 166). Paul used similar strategies of alienation to normalise infertility when asked about his diagnosis.

> Paul: In the case of insemination, the diagnosis was that actually both partners function properly, but that the passage does not work out. It's not a physical diagnosis.

Normalisation strategies also came up in the narratives about ARTs. My interviewees minimised their role and emphasised the normality of conception.

> Sabine: If we wish to have a second child and it does not work out again within a certain time span, then yes, why not [a second ART trial]. To me, it was a small intervention, exactly like the years before when I took the pill, which also were hormones.

At the beginning, Linda had difficulties in normalising insemination and in visualising herself in the role of an infertility patient. After having started the treatment she reported a change of mind towards insemination. Normalisation was seen as necessary to overcome the painful uncertainty regarding a future pregnancy. Circumstances and inconveniences of the ART programme that would not be accepted in other areas of life are normalised. The strong wish for a child at the back of their minds made it possible for my interviewees to highlight the ease of treatment.

> Linda: I imagined it [inseminations] would be more dramatic. I thought it was like a surgical intervention. I really thought it was a kind of operation, but you know, it was extremely easy and simple. I felt – it didn't feel really unnatural at all. Just a little tube that circumnavigates this [passage to the uterus], this is okay.

Paul's experience presents different characteristics. He did not completely normalise insemination, but was able to accept divergence from the common form of conception.

> Paul: It [production of sperm specimen] is a strange situation, even if you can do it at home. The conception occurred kind of shifted on the time axis. The day of the insemination I had to be there [in the clinic] very early, at 7.00 or 7.30 a.m. to hand it in. I therefore had to get up very early while Linda was able to sleep longer (…) it was awkwardly postponed (…). By the time she had the insemination I was already in the office.

Also, non-medical areas and treatments were affected by normalising and relativising efforts. The range of actions so influenced is wide and includes abandonment of alcohol, consultation of an esoteric healer or the discussion of tolerated extra-marital sex to achieve conception. This latter way to a natural conception was proposed by Enzo but suddenly rejected by Janine.

> Enzo: I thought that she [Janine] could have solved the problem much more easily. She is not to blame [it is a male infertility factor], and therefore it crossed my mind that she could just have sex with another man and then she could get pregnant. That sometimes was in the back of my head. Not as fear, but as possibility.

Unlike her husband, Janine could not imagine having a baby with another man or with another man's sperm. Whereas Enzo stressed the naturalness of conception in such an arrangement, Janine preferred natural conception with respect to the biogenetic relation between parents and their children-to-be. She articulated this explicitly later, when talking about donor insemination. Moreover, her repulsion corresponds to contemporary social norms that disapprove of choosing to have a child born out of wedlock that is not genetically related to both parents. In addition, Enzo's offer has to be seen as a sign of desperation or sense of guilt because his sperm was of poor quality. This kind of anticipated self-disposition to suffer cannot be accepted by Janine, culturally and socially, and does not correspond to the cultural ideal of a loving and caring wife and a capable mother-to-be in general. She treats Enzo's suggestion as an absurd idea and both she and her husband try instead to make sense of, or normalise, their conception difficulties.

Most normalisation strategies were pursued with the objective of representing the artificiality of a medical procedure as natural, and can therefore also be classified as naturalisation processes. This is also because infertility patients are often confronted in their social surroundings – in media representations, for example – with the dichotomy of artificial vs. natural (Schröder 2003: 184).

> Alessandra: I suddenly was bothered by the notion 'artificial'. I wondered why it was called 'artificial'. (…) It is only mummy and daddy, there is nothing alien or external in-between.

Many informants were not bothered by this term because they were already accustomed to it from other areas of their life.

> Cyril: My job, everything I do is artificial teeth. For me that is – well everything that renders my wife pregnant and makes her able to give birth to a child has nothing to do with 'artificial'.

My interviewees dissociated themselves from the artificiality of the chosen ARTs by stressing the simplicity of their method or the diffusion of artificial procedures in everyday life, respectively. Applying these strategies, ARTs came to appear quite normal and became an essential part of flexible (reproductive) biographies (e.g. through the use of contraceptives) which are quite positively connoted and widespread in our society (Hess 2008). While pretending not to pay attention to the verdict of third parties who judge their form of reproduction as artificial, interviewees' actions include a paradox in terms, that is to say, non-disclosure of their use of ARTs. This contradiction must not necessarily be considered a stable condition, but could also be interpreted as the first step of normalisation that, above all, had to be performed with regard to their own convictions.

With reference to reproductive treatment, normalisation strategies also originated from the clinic. Enzo and Paul both stress the importance that was attributed to correct labelling on the sperm specimen nameplates. This concern originates from a fear of mixing up 'wrong' genetic substances in a situation where the provenance of the reunited genetic substances is of great importance. Another normalisation effort that derives from the medical setting is the selection of appropriate patient couples and the careful control of suitable behaviour in the site.

> Janine: They [clinic staff] used to ask: 'Oh, have you come alone?' I answered that I didn't need anybody; it's not a big thing. And once (...), Enzo was too early [and therefore already present when Janine had the egg cell puncture] and they suddenly grabbed him and dressed him in a green surgical overall and told him to accompany me.

Thompson also describes this phenomenon in American fertility clinics and interprets it as part of a complex of norms that arise around appropriate, gender specific comportment.

> When there was no male-factor diagnosis, men were expected to accompany their partners at appointments and at several clinics were praised for solicitous behaviour. (...) The norm that male patients ought to manifest as committed and supportive partners was not only present but prescriptive in the site. (Thompson 2005: 133-135)

I would like to emphasise some points regarding normalising and naturalising processes of infertility and ARTs. My informants strove to normalise and naturalise their living conditions with respect to themselves and – in the case of open communication – also within a wider community. This process aimed to integrate their situation as unwillingly childless persons, or as infertility patients, in their biographies and to adjust it according to their ideas about reproduction. Frequently, the course of normalisation included a search for exogenous accounts of infertility, rather than self-inflicted blame, which comprised justifications for treatments and minimisation of the technical aspects. The chosen ARTs are viewed as a small support, as giving nature a helping hand, but not as a complete replacement of nature or an extraordinary mechanisation of formerly pure, natural areas of life. The artificiality of these technologies is diminished and simplicity is stressed, although many informants stated indifference regarding classification of their particular ART experience as artificial. Nevertheless, they knew about public scepticism concerning artificial, scientific reproduction and avoided disclosures. Social norms and meanings are also present when the medical staff exercise control regarding the appropriateness of infertility patients and force couples to perform normatively to comply with the behavioural requirements of future parents.

Conclusion

As it turned out, my informants passed through several stages of reorientation. This process was induced by the detection of infertility and subsequent biographical crisis. Reorientation included integration and acceptance of their changed life situation, reconsideration of 'old' ideas about procreation, and a reestablishment of shifted borders within their biographies. To a great extent, adjustments were oriented around gender and class specific normal biographies (Levy 1977), according to which having children is seen as part of a putatively normal and natural life trajectory. Assisted reproductive technologies hold the potential to fulfil the dream of a family with genetically related offspring – a situation which puts adoption at the second place. Normalisation encompasses processes of integration, acceptance, and relativisation of facts of life that have been taken for granted for a long time. Sometimes, these processes are organised around old norms and values, for example, the idea that both partners had to be present during 'reproduction', or different stages of ARTs. Sometimes they were defined in innovative ways, such as the acceptance of the 'artificial' creation of one's child. In many cases, these strategies are directed towards principles of 'nature' and the definition of what is natural is expanded generously. Franklin (1997: 188) emphasises an 'infamous plasticity of ideas about 'the natural'' with respect to IVF, which also shows up in the quotations from interviewees, particularly with respect to insemination, which was not really regarded as an intervention in natural processes.

At the beginning of what I called 'social normalisation,' my informants had to decide about disclosure. The barrier in communication is noteworthy; most of my informants practised at least partial non-disclosure about their situation. The reasons for this decision varied: shame, the intimacy of the theme; respect for an (infertile) partner; and fear of insensitive reactions were mentioned. In cases where respondents decided upon open discussion, reactions received were generally good, taking the form of empathy or narration of similar cases. This could be interpreted as a sign of rising acceptance of ARTs and as a reduction of related taboos. Some of my informants were convinced that normalcy would come without saying. As future generations probably will treat ARTs just as 'another form of conception' (Becker 2000: 19), these parents plan to inform their child about his or her 'creation'.

Assisted reproduction technologies not only open up new possibilities for involuntarily childless persons, but also prepare grounds for the creation of kinship where traditional beliefs about biological relations must be abandoned. Therefore, everybody is affected and new social forms of dealing with ARTs must be found. Normalisation strategies related to infertility and reproductive treatment prove to be multifaceted and highly adaptive to different situations. They illustrate the struggles of infertile persons with cultural ideologies such as biological parenthood as well as their efforts to fit into the dominating norms of society. Although some might not share interviewees' opinions on the constitution of normality in a given situation, there exists 'a huge overlap in how people in the same society define normalcy' (Becker 2000: 34). For a reader with the same, or similar, cultural background, the rationales and actions of my interviewees may appear plausible and reasonable in most instances.

References

Becker, G. (2000) *The elusive embryo: How women and men approach new reproductive technologies.* Berkeley: University of California Press.

Bundesamt für Statistik (BFS) (2006) Statistik der medizinisch unterstützten Fortpflanzung. *BFS Aktuell 14: Gesundheit.*

de Jong, W. (2008) Intimität auf dem Prüfstand: Neue Verwandtschaftsverhältnisse durch assistierte Reproduktionstechnologien, in Egli, W. and Tomkowiak, I. (Hg.). *Intimität.* Zürich: Chronos Verlag: 137-154.

Fortpflanzungsmedizingesetz (FMedG) Bundesgesetz über die medizinisch unterstützte Fortpflanzung (2006), vom 18. Dezember 1998. SR 810.11.

Franklin, S. (1997) *Embodied Progress: A Cultural Account of Assisted Conception.* London, New York: Routledge.

Franklin, S. (1998) Making miracles: scientific process and the facts of life, in Franklin, S. and Ragoné, H. (eds) *Reproducing Reproduction: Kinship, Power and Technological Innovation.* Philadelphia: University of Pennsylvania Press: 102-117.

Giddens, A. (1991) *The Consequences of Modernity.* Cambridge: Polity Press.

Ginsburg, F.D. and Rapp, R. (1995) *Conceiving the New World Order: The Global Politics of Reproduction.* Berkeley: University of California Press.

Greil, A.L. et al. (1988) Infertility: his and hers, *Gender and Society,* 2 (2): 172-199.

Hadolt, B. (2003) *Kinder-Machen: Eine ethnographische Untersuchung zur Handhabe von ungewollter Kinderlosigkeit und den Neuen Reproduktionstechnologien durch betroffene Frauen und Männer in Österreich.* Verfasst gemeinsam mit Mag. Monika Lengauer. Dissertation an der Fakultät für Human- und Sozialwissenschaften der Universität Göttingen.

Hager, M. (2006) *Kinderwunschlos glücklich? Gewollt kinderlose Akademikerinnen. Eine qualitative empirische Studie zu Lebenssituation und Zukunftsplanung österreichischer Akademikerinnen.* Berlin, Hamburg, Münster: LIT Verlag.

Hess, S. (2008) Der Planungswille zum Kind, *Gen-ethisches Netzwerk.* http://www.gen-ethischesnetzwerk.de/gid/186/thema/hess/ planungswille-zum-kind (last accessed May 19, 2008)

Hirsch, E. ([1993] 1999) Negotiated limits: interviews in South-East England, in J. Edwards, S. Franklin, E. Hirsch, F. Pine and M. Strathern *Technologies of Procreation: Kinship in the Age of Assisted Conception*, London, New York: Routledge: 91-121.

Hohl, M.K. (2003) Aktueller Stand der Fortpflanzungsmedizin in der Schweiz, *Schweizerisches Medizinisches Forum,* 16: 382-386.

Kohler Riessmann, C. (2002) Positioning gender identity in narratives of infertility: South Indian women's lives in context, in Inhorn, M.C. and van Balen, F (eds) *Infertility Around the Globe: New Thinking on Childlessness, Gender and Reproductive Technologies.* Berkeley, Los Angeles, London: University of California Press: 152-171.

Knecht, M. (2003) Die Politik der Verwandtschaft neu denken. Perspektiven der Kultur- und Sozialanthropologie. *Warum noch Familie? Bulletin Texte,* 26. Zentrum für transdisziplinäre Geschlechterstudien der Humboldt-Universität zu Berlin: 52-70.

Johnson, M. (1999) A biomedical perspective of parenthood, in Bainham, A., Day Sclater, S. and Richards, M. (eds) *What Is a Parent? A Socio-Legal Analysis*. Oxford, Portland, Oregon: Hart Publishing: 47-72.

Levy, R. (1977) *Der Lebenslauf als Statusbiographie. Die weibliche Normalbiographie in makrosoziologischer Perspektive.* Stuttgart: Enke.

Mentor, S. (1998) Witches, nurses, midwives and cyborgs: IVF, ART, and agency in the world of technobirth. In: Davis-Floyd, R. and Dumit, J. (eds) *Cyborg Babies: From Techno-Sex to Techno-Tots.* New York: Routledge: 67 – 89.

Onnen-Isemann, C. (2000) Ungewollte Kinderlosigkeit und die Auswirkungen der Reproduktionsmedizin: Der Fall Deutschland, *Forum Qualitative Sozialforschung/Forum: Qualitative Social Research (Online Journal):* 1(1). http://qualitative-research.net/fqs (last accessed July 24, 2007).

Thomspon, Ch. (2005) *Making Parents. The Ontological Choreography of Reproductive Technologies*. Massachusetts: MIT Press.

Schaad, Z. (2008) *Enlich Eltern: Wie Infertilitätserfahrungen und Reproduktionstechnologien den Weg zum ersten Kind prägen. Eine ethnologische Betrachtung.* Unveröffentlichte Lizentiatsarbeit. Zürich: Ethnologisches Seminar.

Schröder, I. (2003) *Die kulturelle Konstruktion von Verwandtschaft unter den Bedingungen der Reproduktionstechnologien in Deutschland.* Dissertation an der sozialwissenschaftlichen Fakultät der Universität Göttingen.

Strathern, M. (1999) Regulation, substitution and possibility. In: Edwards, Jeanette et al. *Technologies of Procreation: Kinship in the Age of Assisted Conception.* London, New York: Routledge: 171-202.

Strathern, M. (2001) Gender: eine Frage des Vergleiches. In: Davis-Sulikowski, Ulrike et al. (Hg.). *Körper, Religion und Macht: Sozialanthropologie der Geschlechterbeziehungen.* Frankfurt a. M.: Campus: 359-393.

Making family and unmaking kin in the Russian media: reproductive technologies and relatedness

Olga Tkach

Assisted reproductive technologies (ARTs) cover a wide range of biotechnological procedures, including determining biological fatherhood and the sex of an unborn child. This study deals with perhaps the most well-known application of ARTs: procedures providing treatment, or assistance, for infertile people wishing to have a baby. These technologies not only create new persons, but also new relationships (Franklin 1999: 162), extending or modifying meanings of kinship, parenthood and family that are usually taken for granted. A range of contemporary American and European research examines how assisted reproductive technologies affect concepts, attitudes and practices in the realm of parenthood and kinship, particularly with respect to social and historical contexts (Cussins 1998; Franklin 1999; Ragoné 1996, 2004; Stone 2000, 2001; Strathern 1991, 1992, 1995; Thompson 2005). This chapter investigates the influence of ARTs on conceptions of relatedness as reflected in Russian public discourse, specifically, mainstream newspapers.

The normative model of the Russian family is a nuclear family, consisting of parents, mother and father, with one or two children who have blood ties with their parents. This type of family is actively promoted by contemporary national policy-makers[1] and is, therefore, part of media discourse. Although various types of parenthood and families are widespread in Russia – adoptive parents, single parents, families having many children – 'new' family and kinship bonds created by the application of ARTs rarely appear in public discussions. The possibilities and outcomes of new reproductive procedures are still problematic for many Russians. These technologies put even the most basic kinship concepts, such as motherhood, in question: is motherhood a genetic relation or one earned through the carrying and delivery of the child? Similarly, fatherhood becomes problematic: is an anonymous sperm-donor a father or just a creator of genetic material? In this chapter, I analyse conceptions of parenthood, kinship and family as reflected in the texts of two Russian national newspapers with large readerships. I will begin with a description of the research data, method and analytical approach, and then explore how kin, parenthood and family relations are established and disambiguated in the newspapers; and the main strategies actors use to 'incorporate 'new data' into pre-existing procedures and objects' (Thompson 2005: 80).

Research data, method and analytical approach

The sample consisted of approximately seventy articles published between 1996 and 2006 in the *Rossiiskaia Gazeta* (RG), Russian Newspaper, and *Argumenty i Fakty* (AiF), Arguments and Facts. Almost all these articles discuss kinship as effected by ARTs and related issues. Applying discourse analysis, I looked for and analysed how actors articulated, explained, evaluated, categorised and interpreted kinship and relatedness as modified by ARTs.[2] These articles are mostly focused interviews with experts in various fields, shedding light on unfamiliar social phenomena related to ARTs, which are sometimes presented in an attempt to shock or astonish readers. Analysis of these articles revealed that experts explaining concepts of family and relatedness are usually journalists, medical doctors, psychologists or lawyers. These are the intermediaries who interpret and explain details related to ARTs, who 'normalize and domesticate procedures' (Thompson 2005: 141). To complement these professionals' weighty opinions, the authors of such articles usually present stories of ordinary people, predominantly couples, of Russian and foreign origin. These examples illustrate the complexity of using ARTs and point out the challenges people face.

People who decide to use ARTs have to involve others in the procedure of conception.[3] Kinship ties become blurred when external genetic material is incorporated in the procreation process. Theoretically, the couple's relationships with donors can be characterised as dispersed kinship, which includes those who have a desire to have a baby, a couple or a single person; and those who assist, clinicians, donors and surrogate mothers (Strathern 1995: 346-363). This analytical differentiation is possible because motherhood and fatherhood are dispersed due to the involvement of a donor in the procreation process. Anthropologists have suggested that kinship connects two domains: the order of nature, represented by genetic or biological kinship; and the order of law, indicating legal kinship (Schneider 1972: 26; Strathern 1992: 17).[4]

The main themes in the analysed texts, which interact and form a 'new' concept of family while problematising it at the same time, are genetic, or biological, and legal relatedness. The actors represented in the articles apply different discursive strategies to legitimise assisted reproduction and dispersed kinship, to normalise these processes and relations. Charis Thompson (2005:81) distinguishes two major means of normalisation: naturalisation and routinisation. Naturalisation refers to how aspects of the situation are rendered as unproblematic or self-evident in the sense of seeming natural, while routinisation refers to how practices and notions are stabilised and fixed in everyday life.[5] How normalisation occurs depends on the stage at which ARTs are applied. Analysis of these texts allows a distinction to be made between two separate steps carried out by a couple: looking for a donor, and preparation for pregnancy; and giving birth and the short period afterwards.[6] Pregnancy is not focused on as a specific stage. Occasionally, it is a topic of discussion with regard to surrogate motherhood. At the first stage, normalisation means making something normal, while at the second stage it means making normative.

Recruiting donors: married couples as key actors

Use of ARTs is represented in Russian newspapers as a project, a deliberate choice made by a heterosexual married couple of reproductive age who have severe fertility problems.[7] A childless couple is seen as a deprived, defective family that hopes to obtain a child. Reproductive technologies are normalised and approved as a welcome remedy for infertility, as a way to solve an individual's or a couple's problems, while also solving the national problem of population decline.[8] The main alternative to ARTs considered in these texts is adoption. Couples featured in these articles view the adoption process as a resource that is unable to provide them with a biological child, genetically linked to at least one of the parents. Moreover, adoption is seen as being available at any time, since it does not strictly depend on the ages of prospective parents.

In order to succeed in conceiving a baby and giving birth, a childless couple must stretch the boundaries of family and kinship at short notice by selecting and recruiting donors.[9] Donors can be anonymous or, alternatively, acquaintances or relatives. Donation of biomaterials can be mapped in complicated cases that involve egg donation by a friend, intergenerational or intrafamilial egg donation, and family-member or commercial surrogates. The most widespread programs described in the texts are artificial insemination (AI), in vitro fertilisation (IVF), egg donation and surrogate motherhood. Each kind of donation creates its own debates about kinship, requiring new ways to re-define, disambiguate and prove parenthood. There are several cases encompassing the most prominent variants of donation programs which reflect different patterns of justifying motherhood and fatherhood as constructed in public discourse.

The 'invisible third': sperm donation and fatherhood

According to the Russian Ministry of Health's decree 'On the use of ARTs in the treatment of female and male infertility' (26.02.2003), a husband's or a donor's sperm can be used in IVF procedure.[10] Stories about anonymous sperm-donors predominate in the newspaper texts.[11] Sperm donation divides fatherhood not only into two separate aspects, but into two personalities. In kinship debates, they do not overlap or even compete with each other. On the one hand, a child has a 'real' genetic father, though the father is absent, as the child will never find and see him; on the other hand, his social father is not 'real'. 'Real' fatherhood is defined as genetic, whereas a social (adoptive) father is second-rate, since he is infertile. Stories about social fatherhood resulting from failed masculinity depict social fathers as indifferent or even malicious. Sometimes a social father abuses a child, or tries to compensate for his inferiority. Therefore, genetic links entail positive and negative emotional bonds between children and parents. It seems that such a child does not have a father at all, either genetic or social.[12] There are a variety of means used to achieve naturalisation, including and excluding both absent genetic fathers and present social fathers. In the newspaper articles I distinguished at least six strategies of normalisation, in the sense of the naturalisation of an absent father, meaning an anonymous genetic donor.

The first strategy is illustrated in the choosing of a donor who is described in the newspaper as looking physically similar to the potential adoptive father, who is usually the female patient's husband. This selection approach demonstrates a genetic priority in determining fatherhood. Thus, social and genetic fatherhood merge. Social fatherhood is symbolically turned into genetic fatherhood.

The second strategy describes a donor who, although never seen, is expected to feel his engagement in the process of making a baby. He is pictured not as an anonymous donor, producing sperm for money, but as someone responsible for his socially useful activity, thinking of his genetic kids, missing them and being spiritually connected to them:

> Besides psychological preparation, it would be better to give a male donor the following piece of advice: when you pass by a boy in the street, pat him on the head. What if he is your son? (RG 16.12.2003)

Although a donor is imagined as a father, he is freed from real responsibility by his anonymity.

The third strategy for normalising absent genetic fathers is found in stories about girls and boys who suddenly discover the circumstances of their conception and attempt to look for their 'real' fathers, though in vain. The genetic father is again regarded as the primary father, the one who is somewhere close. This fantasy supports the idea of blood ties as predominant in defining fatherhood. However, sometimes these stories are interpreted as typical and normal for any teenagers who might seek their genetic identities or personalities.

The fourth strategy refers to ritualisation of an absent, virtual fatherhood by reference to cultural myths rooted in everyday life. Historical determinism or primordialism traces the problem of misidentified fatherhood from ancient times, and marks it as common to all types of societies. According to experts from the groups described above, the issue of the absent, unknown genetic father should not be treated as a tragedy, but as a normal episode that might happen in the life of any family.

> Formerly people had such forms of intimate life that a father was not identified at all. Fatherhood was not so special; it was a rather formal category in many primitive beliefs. Therefore the myth of 'belonging to an indirect father' was embedded in our consciousness. From this all the sentimental literature and soup operas follow, where a supposedly lost, abandoned child is looking for his parents. (AiF 3.02.1999)

The fifth strategy of normalising conception using donated sperm involves postponed parenthood, the preservation of one's own sperm (or eggs) for future use. This message pretends to solve the problem of the donor's anonymity, and it supports the overlapping of genetic and social parenthood as a socially expected result of creating a nuclear family. The genetic materials obtained from future parents are represented as independent actors, potential successors of the family. Genetic kinship is also important in this situation: eggs and sperm donated by relatives and then preserved become significant actors in the system of relatedness.

> People having dangerous jobs – firefighters, military, and policemen – should think of preserving their sperm. Women also have something to freeze – ovum. So when they have problems with ovulation, necessary biomaterial (their own, not donated!) is on hand. (AiF 31.05.2006)

The sixth strategy is targeted at normalisation of assisted genetic fatherhood, by comparing AI and IVF with adoption, and arguing in favour of the former. Unlike adoption, AI and IVF, especially with the sperm of a husband, entail genetic inheritance and reproduce an existing relative. Therefore, such results are more predictable.

> For childless married couples, an ampoule with sperm is a great alternative – infinitely better than the marathon of adoption. Test tube children are always desired. Moreover, they are half one's own. As doctors say, these children are completely genetically healthy, since only healthy men are selected as donors based on all medical requirements, and all ancestors, including grandparents, are examined. Mental health is given extremely close attention when choosing a donor. (RG 27.09.2002)

Justification of the use of donated sperm to create a complete family with a child derives from a genetic view of the world. The genetic approach reflects the simple idea that one person passes on certain characteristics to another person, like a piece of property. In general, genetic fatherhood is perceived as the basic type of fatherhood. Therefore, the figure of a sperm donor is the key to defining kinship. Genetic fatherhood becomes visible where the donor is an acquaintance or a relative. This can be a husband donating for IVF or a dead relative who has donated in advance. By contrast, if a donor is anonymous, social and genetic fatherhood merge. In this case, the anonymous donor is not marked as a member of the family, but necessarily linked directly to the child. The donor looks like a potential social father, and is considered to think about his kids anyway. By and large, a genetic fatherhood does not disappear, but is re-formatted into social fatherhood, and symbolically coexists with it.

Surrogacy and egg donation: the importance of birth

Surrogacy marks a revolution in the meaning of motherhood. Prior to the emergence of reproductive technologies, the 'figure of the mother provided a natural model for the social construction of the 'natural' facts' (Strathern 1991 quoted by Ragoné 2004: 348). In the past, motherhood was always understood as a unified experience, combining social and biological aspects into one, unlike fatherhood which principally exists with a double identity. Surrogate motherhood 'separates motherhood from pregnancy' (Ragoné 2000: 343), and thereby fragments it (2000: 111).[13] The following section examines two variants of surrogacy and understandings of relatedness shown in the analysed texts.

According to the Russian Ministry of Health's decree, 'On the use of ARTs in the treatment of female and male infertility' (26.02.2003), oocytes can be donated by relatives, friends and anonymous donors (RG 6.05.2003).

> The future mother takes an egg from another woman, which is then fertilised by her husband's sperm. Although genetically this baby is not her own, she will be carrying it for nine months by herself. (AiF 19.03.1997)

In this case, the process of carrying a baby normalises the odd situation of using a donated egg. In egg donation, the genetic mother has no rights.[14] Motherhood is not defined in genetic terms, rather in terms of carrying and giving birth.[15]

Inability to conceive a baby is dealt with by searching among relatives or acquaintances for a genetic mother.[16] As a rule, egg donation draws on the resources of the multigenerational family. Through recruiting relatives from different generations as donors, kinship is rearranged and intergenerational hierarchies and boundaries are mixed up:

> Olga is 48. This is her second marriage. Olga's husband is much younger, than she. They both want a baby. But the mother's age… (…) Olga's twenty year old daughter agreed to be a donor. The process of artificial insemination passed successfully. Now Olga is pregnant. But how will the family manage to identify kinship relations: who is the mother, who is the sister of this baby? Maybe it doesn't matter? The most important thing is that a child was born. (RG 9.01.1998)

The author of this quotation is disoriented by shifts in generational hierarchies and obligations, and does not even want to figure out the configurations of kinship in this entangled case. Surrogacy is represented as assistance or help, and is described using language categorised as appropriate for intimate and friendly relationships. The donation of an egg is not problematised with regard to kinship in these newspaper texts, and the motherhood rights accruing to the donating woman are not negotiated. The donor simply helps her close friend or relative by providing genetic material as a gift, which is then privatised through the process of giving birth. The means of naturalisation of egg donation is biologisation: it does not matter who is genetically linked to the child, it only matters who gives birth.

Secondary or alien moms? Between commodification and altruistic help

The boundary between help and paid service is regarded as more prominent in the case of surrogate motherhood – an official program under Russian Family Law. According to this legislation, only married couples with severe fertility problems can apply to hire a surrogate mother. It is strictly prohibited for healthy and fertile couples 'to avoid pregnancy and the painful process of giving birth'. Only the medical aspects of the procedure are regulated. The rest of the problems, such as legalisation of a baby by genetic parents or financial and emotional relationships between both parties, are not dealt with by the law and are negotiated by the genetic parents and the surrogate mother personally. Verbal agreements between surrogate mothers and couples prevail, although written contracts are also sometimes made.

With regard to the United States in the 1960s, David Schneider (1968 as quoted by Ragoné 2004: 343) points out that 'the social mother is similar to an adoptive mother in that her relationship to the child exists not in nature, but in law alone'. I assume that in the case of surrogate motherhood, this link is not evident. At first glance, as in the case of the other procedures, it is the couple that chooses surrogate motherhood. However, surrogacy may become completely a project of the social mother, in which she makes a last effort at producing a baby. Prior to adoption, the social mother has an arduous journey, including looking for a surrogate mother, negotiating with her the rules of behaviour, creating healthy conditions for her to bear the baby and managing emotional tensions. This program bonds a surrogate mother with a future social mother rather than a future father. It merges the adoptive mother and the surrogate mother into one in order to maintain the unity of experience. It erases their boundaries (Ragoné 2004: 353).

Women performing the role of a surrogate mother are usually depicted in these newspaper articles as single mothers or mothers from a family with financial problems. The candidates are strongly required to be between 25 and 35 years of age and to have their own healthy children. The surrogate mother's personal characteristics are restricted by the couples to her ability to bear a child. She should be touched by the parents' situation, but not in touch with a baby which, by agreement, is not hers. In many cases, parents prefer not to delegate the selection of donors to the medical system or other professionals.[17] One patient shares her experience of searching for a surrogate mother:

> My husband and I were engaged in choosing a mother for our children for a long period of time. We met some of them at the Institute [the renowned D.I. Otto Institute of Genealogy in St.Petersburg], but we didn't trust them at all. They asked for extremely large sums of money for their services, and it seemed to us that they would rather take care of their pockets than of our babies. Olga is not from the Institute at all. I knew her for a long time, though not very well. She has two children, and I've seen how she treats them. Therefore, I had no doubt that she will also conscientiously bear my babies. By the way, her cost for the 'service' suited us. (RG 8.06.2002)

Recent literature on surrogate motherhood often divides the strategies of surrogates into two groups. For instance, Melissa Lane makes a distinction 'between 'contract' surrogacy in which a formal contract for some consideration is involved, and 'gift' surrogacy where relatives, friends or acquaintances arrange surrogacy as non-financial and non-contractual relationship among themselves' (Lane 2003: 121; Ragoné 2003; Blyth and Potter 2003). 'The 'natural' can be linked to kinship and gift as contrasted with the contractual – for example, familial surrogacy versus contractual surrogacy' (Lane 2003: 125). This division is also confirmed by the data analysed here. However, willingness to help and commercial interest are deeply interrelated and overlap in the practice of surrogacy. Therefore, the terms second mom, revealing the perspective of altruistic help, versus alien mom, proving an idea of a calculating market actor, describe the two faces of a surrogate mother which alternate in the texts.

The first aspect of surrogate motherhood is friendly support, or help, provided by a hired woman. A surrogate mother is depicted as giving birth to a baby 'for a sister', 'for a friend', generally for another woman, but not for a couple or a family. Doctors actively support this idea. 'The patients are basically relatives or friends of genetic parents. They run risks of surrogacy being inspired by pure altruism, not by money.' (AiF 15.11.2000)

> The mother gave birth to the babies for her childless sister. Officially she became a surrogate mother to help her relative and also to cope with her own financial troubles, since she is a single mother with two children. The sister and her husband are wealthy people, but they do not have children. Close relatives are extremely welcome in surrogate motherhood programs. [...] According to the rules of surrogate motherhood, both women are going to the maternity hospital, and then the genetic mother leaves it with a baby. (RG 21.02.2006)

Although surrogacy by acquaintances is sometimes preferred by couples, there are few narratives about it in these newspaper articles. The prevalence of stories about non-relative surrogate mothers might be considered as a way to normalise breaks with the social order. The level of emotional closeness between social and biological moms normalises the artificial fragmentation of motherhood. In the stories presented in these articles, surrogate mothers are expected to have certain moral qualities, besides their physical state. The surrogate is basically moved by the misfortune of unsuccessful parents, while the only obligation of a sperm-donor, is to be invisible and stay away from the family that uses his donated genetic material.

Individuals identified in the newspaper articles as experts on ARTs, predominantly doctors, attempt to refute the substitution of emotional and biological closeness between the two moms and, correspondingly, of a surrogate mother and child. They prove that a baby does not inherit any genetic traits from a surrogate mother. The only way a surrogate can influence a fetus is through improper behaviour during the child-bearing period. Therefore, the rules of a surrogate mother's behaviour are negotiated with the social parents before the start of the procedure to reduce possible harm. The naturalness of a surrogate's services during the pregnancy period is interpreted as 'the real work of mothering the birth mother does' (Lane 2003: 125). Surrogate motherhood is contracted by both sides as a sacrifice for a planned baby, therefore it is legitimate. Later on, adoptive mothers deemphasise the importance of biological relatedness of a child to a mother, giving a priority to genetic motherhood.

> Olga is carrying twins for Tatiana. 'Aren't you embarrassed, these babies are not yours?' I [the journalist] ask Tatiana.
> 'What are you talking about? There are definitely created from my cells!' (RG 8.06.2002)

> (…) the surrogate mother is a container. For instance, if you take a duck's egg and put it in a hen's nest, the egg will not hatch a chicken, but a duck. (AiF 25.02.2004)

The second aspect of surrogate motherhood is its role as an expensive commercial service. It is described as an informal, even shadow, market which has hidden dangers. Predominantly, genetic parents are represented as potential victims of a surrogate mother's greediness, which at the same time implicitly competes with her sympathy for a childless couple. In general, the behaviour of surrogates is depicted as unpredictable and uncertain. Stories about surrogate mothers blackmailing couples during pregnancy or afterwards are frequently alluded to in the texts.

The commercial component of surrogate motherhood provokes opponents of surrogacy to criticise this practice, giving a moral priority to adoption. They argue that surrogate children are anyway not the parents' own, they are purchased with money.

> Surrogate motherhood is a caprice of rich people, rolling in money. (…) Does an ordinary family really have such enormous money to buy an 'incubator

> with legs'? (…) if you want a baby (…) adopt an orphan, even better, adopt a couple of them, form an orphanage, then raise and educate the children for these twenty thousand dollars! (AiF 25.02.2004)[18]

Surrogate motherhood actualises the priority of genetic motherhood: Blood relatedness to a child is represented as more important than a biological relationship. By contrast, egg donation emphasises biological motherhood – that is the carrying of a child. A couple gives priority to a domain of kinship that is likely to link a child to a social mother, consuming a service of surrogacy. Surrogate children are normalised via adoption. However, prior to it, surrogacy is routinised by defining it as an act of help, emotional involvement and sympathy, qualities that are widespread within families. Surrogacy is viewed as comparable with organ or blood donation by relatives. In the case of commercial surrogacy, it is normalised by the idea of mutual help (financial support of a woman living in poverty) and the genetic bond of adoptive mother, father and child.

After giving birth: the agenda of Russian Family Law

Assisted reproductive technologies entail the natural facts of procreation being doubly assisted on an institutional level: by technological and medical advances and by legislation (Strathern 1992: 20). After the child is born, Family Law comes into play. It introduces normative boundaries for relations between a newborn child and the parents that have gone through assisted reproductive programs. Agreement to the procedures from both spouses is a legal requirement. The last stage of constructing a new family is adoption. Russian Health Law and Family Law are here the main frameworks for legitimating, regulating and structuring kinship ties created by ARTs. At this stage, donors have disappeared and the relationships between couples and children are reinforced.

Numerous stories about the complex procedure of legalising parenthood through ARTs lead to the conclusion that the multiple genetic and biological links arising from these technologies are very difficult to accommodate in Russia's incomplete and inflexible legislation. Basically, children born thanks to ARTs are legalised through adoption, including proof that all operations were legally provided by specialists in the hospital. Legal registration of children born by means of AI and IVF does not significantly differ from usual practices. Russian legislation maintains that a child born within a marriage following the use of AI or embryo implantation on the basis of a written agreement is to be regarded as the child of the mother and her husband.[19] The most challenging cases in this respect are surrogate motherhood and posthumous conception. The surrogate child is linked to the mother legally, in the same way as to a father. A child born within a marriage after the use of surrogacy on the base of a written agreement is to be regarded as the child of the mother and her husband only if the biological surrogate mother does not recognise the child as hers.[20] The surrogate mother simply makes an official statement that the spouses who hired her are the parents of a child. In the event that she wants to keep the baby, Russian Family Law protects her rights as the legal mother. Current legislation does not cover other variants of surrogacy, except implantation of an embryo conceived from an egg of a future social mother and sperm of a social father. In all other cases, legal registration of the child can present a range of problems.

A special case raising a host of complex ethical and social issues is posthumous conception, or the use of a deceased man's sperm to become pregnant. In the case of posthumous conception, the problem is that the genetic father is truly absent, but biologically present through the use of his gametes. His social presence, as a father and husband, must be actively constructed through the creation of contexts and connections (Strathern 1993 quoted by Simpson 2001: 3). Although cases of posthumous conception are not very common in this data, they tend to be discussed from a legal rather than ethical perspective. The disrupted order of inheritance, as a result of conceiving a child long after the father has died, complicates the legalisation of parenthood. The following quotation illustrates the problem of legalisation of a baby born by a surrogate mother who was hired by the baby's grandma.

The latter managed to preserve her 19 year-old son's sperm since the time before he dies from cancer:

> Ekaterina Germanovna [the grandmother] was greatly surprised when she was told that, according to the law, her baby cannot exist. If his father is dead, he cannot be entered on a birth certificate. The law does not envisage babies of a long deceased parent being born. Neither does it envisage the baby being carried by an absolutely alien woman. They say she who gave birth is the mother. Officials do not care whether she was a surrogate or not. Here Gosha [the new born child] appears to be an alien: he has neither a legal surname, nor a legal father, nor a legal grandmother. (RG 27.01.2006)

Bob Simpson (2001: 10) argues that the prior existence of marriage legitimises subsequent attempts to use posthumous conception which, in turn, forms the basis of a claim to legitimate the issue, justifying kinship ties and inscribing them somehow into existing legislation. Ekaterina Germanovna's son was not married. Lacking a formal basis to justify the newborn child, the grandmother actively insisted on the right of a mother to use her son's cells to conceive a baby. The posthumously conceived child is both the realisation of the father's intent and a repository for the memory of him. Furthermore, with the increasing tendency to stress genetics in the description of relationships, the child will be marked with its father's death in ways which suggest substitution and replication (Simpson 2001: 3). This unique story was reprinted several times and represented as shocking for the audience and challenging for the grandmother. Another description of Gosha's situation was as follows:

> The child was born in a non-standard way and was not covered by the current Russian legislation on the registration of children. He was required to take the surname of the surrogate mother; and registry officials did not want to hear anything about his a long-deceased father. (RG 24.03.2006)

Finally, the grandmother applied for guardianship, so she would be able to adopt the child, Gosha, who was genetically linked to her. Though it could be argued that posthumous conception creates novel or even post-modern kinship; such a position ignores the ways that these innovations are pressed into the service of making and affirming conventional family structures and roles. In the absence of formal statements, reproductive intent can be seen to derive from the strength of conjugal sentiment (Simpson 2001: 3).

Within the frame of ARTs, different relationships between genetic, biological, and social kinship are possible. Usually the concept of kinship, especially parenthood, somehow slides between these variants, and one pattern can be converted into another. Moral aspects of this transformation, which are of great importance when choosing a donor, can compete with the legal aspects in the period after giving a birth. Genetic kinship cannot always be inscribed in legal kinship. An implicit message of these stories is the necessity of improving Russian family legislation, making it more flexible and incorporating different ways of conceiving that reflect the development of new technologies.

Conclusions

In an 'ideal' family, all modes of kinship should be coherent with each other. However, such coherence is often far from reality, especially if this kinship is being constructed by means of ARTs. Different meanings of relatedness depend on the stage at which the procedures and concrete donorship program are applied. Assisted reproductive technologies highlight biogenetic and social domains of kinship. Depending on what types of donation are used, couples choose the type of kinship that they think bonds them, or one of them, to a common child. They re-define very broadly the priority of genetic or legal principles of kinship if it supports their plan. The analysed texts suggest the conclusion that biogenetic kinship takes priority in the private sphere, for the family itself, while legalised ties with a newborn child have to be proved by the bureaucratic authorities and demonstrated in the public sphere. The genetic relationship that exists is regulated by law and, therefore, deproblematised.

A couple is depicted at a crucial stage of their shared biography or history, in their attempts to conceive a baby and to cope with infertility problems. Use of ARTs cover a rather short period in the life of a family, but these technologies can profoundly rearrange social relations with relatives and those who somehow participate – physically or emotionally – in the procedure. I consider these forms of 'assisted' kinship as situational and short-term because, after the successful use of ARTs, their results are inscribed within the framework of the nuclear family by means of private agreements and legislation. Obviously, applying ARTs creates a clear asymmetry in the genetic links of a child to both parents. However, the fact that only one of the parents is genetically linked to the child is finally resolved. Regardless of the variety of 'natural' links of a child to a mother and father, this combination is re-arranged into one desirable type of social relations, in particular kin relations of parents and a child. Temporally fragmented fatherhood and motherhood are finally united into general social parenthood. Other participants in the process of conceiving, except social parents, disappear from the texts. From a moral perspective, ARTs are normalised by describing a married couple coping with its fertility problems as socially responsible and successful in reproducing a complete family at all costs. Therefore, the resulting children are extremely desired by the parents, and 'naturally' born, not adopted. The final version is inscribed in the 'ideal' image of the nuclear family with children. Moreover, this family is represented as exemplary in terms of special atmosphere of closeness between children and their parents, who made a lot of efforts to have a baby.

Assisted reproductive technologies have introduced into regular parlance the distinction between social and biological parenthood (Strathern 1992: 19). The actors in these newspaper articles are trying to get used to these new terms and introduce their own terms. This explains the logic of the procedures to the audience through terms like 'bio-mother', 'bio-father', 'second mother' and 'alien mother'. In other words, the newspaper articles provide their readers with information about the diversity of opportunities and challenges created by ARTs, including different configurations of relatedness they generate. However, as Strathern (1995: 353) points out:

> (…) 'more' kinship does not necessarily lead to 'more' relatives. (…) not all biogenetic relationships may be activated as social ones.

In these newspaper articles, ARTs do not disrupt normative ideas about family and kinship. On the contrary, efforts are made to preserve the cultural notions of 'real' biological parenthood and nuclear family. We might expect that ARTs have the potential to liberate family roles and kinship ties; but, in this context, discussion and exploration of these issues reinforces the nuclear family in Russian public discourse, overshadowing the great variability of postmodern family forms that exist in contemporary Russian society, including single-parent families and child-free couples.

Notes

[1] See the 'Conception of the Demographic Development of Russian Federation until 2015' in Declaration of the Government of the Russian Federation, June 3, 2005: http://www.minzdravsoc.ru/docs/government/rasp/9 (last accessed July 22, 2009).

[2] In conducting textual analysis, I used the following tools. First, I asked what kinds of repertoires are available, possible, and legitimate in the Russian social context? Second, I examined which issues actors link together or separate; what kinds of distinctions they make and how; their representation of interrelationships between different entities (for example between active kinship and anonymity; artificial and natural fertilisation; surrogacy and adoption; and commodification or assistance in surrogacy). Third, I paid attention to intertextuality in the data by exploring how concepts and meanings are circulated, re-coded and transferred to new contexts; how actors draw elements from economic, ethical, juridical or family discourse and embed them in new contexts.

[3] The most widespread procedures and techniques used are artificial insemination (AI); in vitro fertilisation (IVF); egg (oocyte) donation; fetus donation; and surrogate motherhood. Male donors contribute sperm; female donors contribute eggs and fetuses.

[4] Unlike adoption, which is legally framed and organised, use of ARTs presupposes a complicated combination, or even conflict, between two different orders. Based on the idea of fragmentation of parenthood and the variety of practices people can perform in the process of 'making a baby', Robert Snowden and his

colleagues propose up to ten different terms to cover the concepts of 'mother' and 'father', including genetic mother, carrying mother, nurturing mother, complete mother (covering the stages of conception, gestation and care for a child), genetic father, and complete father (Snowden et al. 1983 quoted by Stone 2000: 292).

[5] According to Thompson (2005:12), normalisation includes routinisation, primarily in terms of skilled local knowledge exercised by medical personnel and patients in conjunction with medical technologies. Medical personnel possess routinised skills that implicate the enactment of epistemic norms of seeing, feeling, and knowing, according to a certain division of labour, such as reading ultrasound scans or carrying out pelvic exams (see also de Jong, this volume).

[6] There are almost no episodes dealing with how children learn about the circumstances of their origins and their ensuing actions. There were several references to foreign newspaper articles about children searching for a genetic father, though these belonged to the first two or three years of the period analysed. The articles do not contain any examples or discussion of long-term social effects. Assisted reproductive technologies are reduced to a very limited activity aimed at conceiving and giving birth. The remaining issues related to bringing up children – their genetic background, the possible influence of inherited diseases, children's right to know the circumstances of their origin, problems with their family identity and possible conflicts – are obscured.

[7] Infertility entails not only a medical, but also a social diagnosis, which is described using alarmist language, such as a 'fault', a 'sin' of both spouses, a 'tragedy' for the family, and a 'terrible punishment'.

[8] Cases of single women are dealt with very rarely, though such women are officially allowed to use IVF. Lesbian couples applying for such procedures are barely discussed in the texts. The few examples are not represented as 'real stories'. Therefore, singles and lesbians applying for such treatment lack the means of normalisation and grounding in public discourse and, correspondently, in everyday practice.

[9] Relationships between spouses are not emphasised, they are seen as unproblematic. Sometimes this unity is only proclaimed, not actively shown, since a woman is shown as a representative of a couple, talking in the name of the partnership.

[10] Patients choose a donor voluntary and independently, based on the physical and health descriptions (RG, 6.05.2003).

[11] There are no references to persons asked by friends or relatives to donate sperm. I assume this anonymity prevents calling spousal relationship into ques-

tion, allowing a couple to concentrate on conceiving, and avoiding jealousy and suspicion that using an acquaintance as a donor might provoke.

[12] Sex-role stereotyping assigns to males the role of initiators, thus defining infertile men as powerless or passive, and as unable to undertake successfully that which is considered 'appropriate masculine behaviour' (Ragoné 2004: 346), including fatherhood. Lundin (2001: 151) shows that, through IVF, new expectations about sexual competence and new demands on sperm producers are created. There is hardly any reference to older phallocentric values or to modern equality in this context.

[13] Ragoné (2000: 343) distinguishes three categories created by surrogacy: the biological mother, that is the women who contributes the ovum (the woman formerly assumed to be the 'real mother'); the gestational mother, that is the woman who gestates the embryo but bears no genetic relationship to the child; and the social mother, the women who nurtures and raises the child.

[14] Russian Family Law also gives its priority to biological mother as a woman who gave birth to a child (see also Brednikova, Nartova and Tkach, this volume).

[15] In this case, biological means 'carrying' of the child (Stone 2001).

[16] Unlike sperm donation, egg donation is a more delicate operation, requiring a personal approach to a female donor. The technique of organising oocyte banks is not described, while the details and technique of donating sperm and creating sperm banks are widely discussed.

[17] The widespread problem of an institutional credibility gap leads to preference for a personal, reputation-oriented approach in selecting a donor. One might suppose that the lack of formalisation in this sphere contradicts the idea of a donor's anonymity, where the family is safe from the sudden appearance of an acquaintance related to a baby genetically or biologically. Nevertheless, unlike having a child by AI or IVF, surrogacy includes long-term communication. Moreover, the well-being of the bearing mother can directly influence the future child.

[18] Interestingly, unlike discussion on sperm donation, in which adoption is not welcomed, opponents of surrogacy uses adoption as an argument for relatedness of a child to the parents.

[19] Family Law of Russian Federation, Section 4, Chapter 10, article 51.

[20] Family Law of Russian Federation, Section 4, Chapter 10, article 51.

References

Blyth, E. and Potter, C. (2003) Paying for it? Surrogacy, market forces and assisted conception, in R. Cook, Sh. Sclater and F. Kaganas (eds) *Surrogate Motherhood: International Perspectives*. Oxford, Portland, Oregon: HARTS Publishing: 227-242.

Cussins, C. (1998) Producing reproduction: techniques of normalization and naturalization in infertility clinics, in S. Franklin and H. Ragoné (eds) *Reproducing Reproduction: Kinship, Power, and Technological Innovation*. Philadelphia, Pennsylvania: University of Pennsylvania Press: 66-101.

Franklin, S. (1999) Making representations: the parliamentary debate on the human fertilisation and embryology act, in J. Edwards et al. (eds) *Technologies of Procreation: Kinship in the Age of Assisted Conception*. London, New York: Routledge: 127-165.

Lane, M. (2003) Ethical issues in surrogacy arrangements, in R. Cook, Sh. Sclater and F. Kaganas (eds) *Surrogate Motherhood: International Perspectives*. Oxford, Portland, Oregon: HARTS Publishing: 121-139.

Lundin, S. (2001). The threatened sperm: parenthood in the age of biomedicine, in L. Stone (ed) *New Directions in Anthropological Kinship*. Lanham: Rowman and Littlefield: 139-155.

Ragoné, H. (1996) Chasing the blood tie: surrogate mothers, adoptive mothers, and fathers, *American Ethnologist*, 23(2): 352-365.

Ragoné, H. (2000) Of likeness and difference: how race is being transfigured by gestational surrogacy, in H. Ragoné and F.W. Twine (eds) *Ideologies and Technologies of Motherhood: Race, Class, Sexuality, Nationalism*. New York, London: Routledge: 56-75.

Ragoné, H. (2003) The gift of life: surrogate motherhood, gamete donation and construction of altruism, in R. Cook, Sh. Sclater and F. Kaganas (eds) *Surrogate Motherhood: International Perspectives*. Oxford and Portland, Oregon: HARTS Publishing: 209-226.

Ragoné, H. (2004) Surrogate motherhood and American kinship, in R. Parkin and L. Stone (eds) *Kinship and Family: An Anthropological Reader*. Oxford: Blackwell Publishing Ltd.: 342-361.

Schneider, D. (1968) *American Kinship: A Cultural Account*. Englewood Cliffs, N.Y.: Prentice-Hall.

Schneider, D. (1972) What is kinship all about? in P. Reining (ed.) *Kinship Studies in the Morgan Centennial Year*. Washington: Society of Anthropology: 32-63.

Simpson, B. (2001) Making 'bad' deaths 'good': the kinship consequences of posthumous conception, *Journal of the Royal Anthropological Institute*, 7(1): 1-18.

Snowden, R. et al. (1983) *Artificial Reproduction*. London: Allen and Unwin.

Stone, L. (2000) *Kinship and Gender: An Introduction*. Boulder, Colorado, Oxord: Westview Press.

Stone, L. (ed). (2001) *New Directions in Anthropological Kinship*. Lanham: Rowman and Littlefield.

Strathern, M. (1991) *The Pursuit of Certainty: Investigating Kinship in the Late Twentieth Century*. Paper presented at the American Anthropology association Meeting. Chicago, Illinois.

Strathern, M. (1992) *Reproducing the Future: Essays on Anthropology, Kinship and the Assisted Reproductive Technologies*. New York: Routledge.

Strathern, M. (1993) The work of culture: an anthropological sperspective, in A. Clarke and E. Parsons (eds) *Culture, Kinship and Genes*. Houndmills: Macmillan.

Strathern, M. (1995) Displacing knowledge: technology and the consequences for kinship, in F.D. Ginsburg and R. Rapp (eds) *Conceiving the New World Order: The Global Politics of Reproduction*. Berkeley, Los Angeles, London: University of California Press: 346-363.

Thompson, C. (2005) *Making Parents: The Ontological Choreography of Reproductive Technologies*. Cambridge, London: The MIT Press.

Reproductive technologies, embryos and children

Embryos made in Switzerland: surprising persons and relatives

Willemijn de Jong

Anthropological studies show that 'embryo tales' are a rich source for understanding foundational aspects of sociality and cosmology. Swiss embryo tales are no exception. In this article I investigate meanings about embryos that medical and religious experts and lay people create in the Swiss context of assisted reproductive technologies (ARTs), especially in vitro fertilisation (IVF) and related research. I further examine the knowledge practices that are used to normalise the newness of these technologies and their effects on embryos. My study is inspired by work on embryonic personhood; on the embryo as a new kinship entity; and on the normalisation of kinship and gender. My aim is to show that embryos made by ARTs and actors in Switzerland are a surprise, as full persons and relatives, or incipient ones, and they often have a spiritual quality (Strathern 2005).

Lynn Morgan (2003: 289), who has published extensively on reproduction and personhood, argues in her article 'Embryo tales' that 'embryo meanings arise out of historically particular social anxieties and controversies'. Embryos are products of the times and cultural contexts in which they live. For example, embryos in the United States today tell us about the politics of gender, reproduction and the commodification of body parts. Modern visualising technologies, which have proliferated since the 1970s – such as sonography and the images it produces – are crucial in the creation of embryonic or fetal subjects. These technologies enable the assignment of personhood and agency to the unborn and have also become relevant to abortion and reproductive politics. Referring to Morgan (2003), I will analyse in what ways the embryo is imbued with meaning and how 'the beginning of life' (Kaufman and Morgan 2005) is conceptualised in Switzerland in the twenty-first century.

Embryos are a focus of investigation for Sarah Franklin as well (see for example Franklin 2006). Her earlier work (Franklin [1993] 1999) on the meanings of the embryo and kinship in parliamentary debates related to the Human Fertilisation and Embryology Act in Britain around 1990 has been particularly useful for me. Referring to Donna Haraway, Franklin describes embryos as cyborg kinship entities, a new kinship entity that embodies both science and nature. The embryo is also the embodiment of a new kind of kinship, a postmodern one, because it embodies scientific progress and technological potency that displaces earlier assumptions about nature. Moreover, in the context of embryology, 'micro-kinship' is created which is 'composed of unfamiliar kinship entities, germinal matter in need of classification' (Franklin 1999: 161). Following Franklin, I will analyse how the embryo is constituted as a kinship entity and what kind of familiar and unfamiliar kinship it generates in Switzerland.

In her impressive ethnography on ARTs in theUnited States, Charis Thompson (2005) postulates a flexible 'choreography' between the natural and the cultural to achieve normalisation as a reaction to destabilisation of the body and kinship through ARTs, which include possibilities for conservation and innovation. With reference to that research, I analyse what kinds of naturalising and socialising strategies experts and lay people use to normalise – and eventually to innovate – relatedness with embryos in the Swiss context of ARTs (see also de Jong, this volume).

I will begin with an examination of selected medical and religious discourses about ARTs and the embryo from Swiss mass media publications that appeared between 2000 and 2007. Embryo tales of medical and religious institutions are of special interest historically and culturally, and they also have important effects on body politics. Then I will analyse the statements of five mothers about ARTs and the embryo from interviews conducted in 2007 with middle-class parents living in the German-speaking part of Switzerland. As I am interested in personal opinions about ARTs in general, in addition to public opinion, people who did not experience IVF were chosen, as in certain studies in Britain (Edwards 1999; Hirsch 1999).[1]

ARTs and embryos made by medical experts

To study public discourses of reproductive medical expertise, I chose a newspaper supplement on ARTs published on the 24 August, 2007 in the *Tages-Anzeiger*, the most wide-spread daily newspaper in German-speaking Switzerland. In English, the supplement is entitled *Infertility: A Guide to the Unfulfilled Wish for a Child*, and was published by Mediaplanet, a company that regularly produces newspaper supplements. The field of ARTs takes on a scientific enlightenment character, sprinkled with spiritual elements of salvation in this publication. The journalistic articles deal specifically with hormones; libido and evolution as a means of explaining gender relations; the vagaries of female reproductive processes; the increasingly poor quality of sperm; promising types of reproductive treatments, with reference to those available abroad; and the hopeful future of molecular genetics. At the same time, commercialisation is clearly evident in advertisements and implicit in certain articles.

Medical treatment is presented as a normal and mostly successful way to 'struggle against childlessness' (2007: 7). Although about seventy percent of couples cannot overcome childlessness through ARTs,[2] this is not mentioned. Only one clinician stressed that the 'baby take home rate' should not be the sole quality criteria of reproductive medicine and recommended counselling and searching for a way of life without a child (2007: 14). In keeping with the positive and salutary image of science in this journalistic biomedical thinking, nature is conceptualised as a negative force which may disturb family planning (2007: 4). Several medical experts obviously use this publication to present opinions on health policies. Some openly contested the reproductive medicine legislation (*Fortpflanzungsmedizingesetz*) that came into force in 2001, by advocating pre-implantation genetic diagnosis (2007: 8). This technique enables physicians to check for genetic defects in 'embryos' in the laboratory on the third day after fertilisation, rather than when pregnancy is already underway and abortion is more problematic. Furthermore, 'reproductive tourism', or visiting other countries for egg donation, is discussed as an accepted fact, at least for heterosexual couples and single women, and is implicitly promoted (2007: 9).

After having looked at the main representations of ARTs, we turn to the meanings given to the embryo in these texts. The term 'embryo' is hardly explicitly mentioned, and when the term appears, it is in relation to other cellular forms or 'germinal matter' (Franklin 2007: 5), such as hormones that stimulates sexuality; egg cells that undergo 'normal aging' which often impedes having a child (2007: 10); and blastocysts with special reproductive potency (2007: 16). The embryo is mostly constructed in a technical and unemotional sense. For example, the final phase of IVF is described thus:

> Developing embryos are finally implanted into the womb of the woman. Possibly the procedure has to be repeated with the woman's own frozen embryos (...) The transfer, i.e. the introduction of the embryos into the womb itself, is a simple procedure without pain (2007: 7-8).

Can we talk about the embryo as a kin entity here? In one article the embryo is emphatically related to love, the 'intimate wish for a child' of the couple, and the anxieties and tensions of partnerships, if this wish is not fulfilled. The director of seven private ART clinics in Europe, one just beyond the Swiss border, has created the slogan, 'Giving Love Life', which is also the title of a one-page advertisement. This fits perfectly with the suggestion that current identities and sexualities in the context of IVF are strongly focused on an asexual, platonic form of intimate love (Bock v. Wülfingen 2006: 12). Moreover, the rhetoric in these articles evokes familiar forms of kinship, parenthood and particularly motherhood:

> 'Just the first time it worked out well,' says the mother with delight. Both parents look happily at their small daughters who are hardly half a year old. They are satisfied, two-egg-twins. (2007: 13)

A kin relation of an unfamiliar kind is implicitly created between the embryo, the clinician, and the mother, when the journalist attests that the director has created a 'very adequate word' for the transfer of an embryo, literally 'return-gift' (*Rückgabe*) (2007: 13). A similar kin relationship is evoked when the journalist talks about a couple from Zurich with a 'sweet, fair baby' who wants to present the child to their IVF doctor, upon which the director comments that 'she [that doctor] finally also produced it [the baby]' (2007: 13). This also shows an additional dimension of hierarchy or power in the making of this unfamiliar kinship, created in the process in which 'nature' was 'helped out' through the assistance of a doctor.

Unfamiliar kinship is created here also in a more comprehensive sense, when the journalist characterises the embryo as a kind of miracle:

> It is hardly believable that in that microscopic, tiny form all the predispositions, the chromosomes, which define the sex, and the whole hereditary material (*Erbgut*) of a human being, are already contained. (2007: 13)

We can call this geneticised kinship, or micro-kinship:

> a simultaneous cellularisation of our origins, identities and inheritances while also making of kinship a universal human connectedness that looks more like the 'family of man.' (Franklin 1999: 161)

Embryos are further presented as future kin entities in prominent photographic images of prospective babies and children who are, in most cases, sweetly posed with their happy-looking parents. A loving but 'infertile' (and thus, sick) heterosexual couple needing treatment and care is the contrasting focus of most of the texts. 'Childlessness is a Sickness' is the title of one of the articles, which can be read as if any mature individual who has no children is ill (2007: 8). Having no children, and thus a lack of intimate kinship, as we can call it, is normalised here as a sickness with which one in six couples must cope, in accordance with the World Health Organization's definition of infertility. Additionally, this sickness is gendered and aged: after the age of thirty-five, female fertility decreases dramatically (2007: 10); but sperm quantity and quality are identified as bigger problems (2007: 6).

In sum, we can say that biomedical discourse normalises and effects the body politic in paradoxical ways. On the one hand, these texts specifically focus on sick reproductive body parts and pursue a hegemonic and normalising discourse by using statistics and a language of medical or biological risk. 'Nature' is rarely presented, and if so, it is presented negatively. These discursive strategies cannot be conflated with naturalisation. They are better denoted as biologisation in the sense that they emphasise biogenetic substance (Schneider 1968). On this level of discourse, potential clients are approached and reassured that having babies is technologically feasible and worthwhile, despite financial costs and stress. On the other hand, the nation-state with its strict legal conditions regarding ARTs is addressed, and contested through the promotion of forbidden procreative technologies. The 'biomedical mode of (re)production' (Thompson 2005) is present in this discourse as an undercurrent. The loss of patients through reproductive tourism and the loss of Switzerland as a site of advanced scientific research are hinted at as threats to the attractiveness of the country on the international market of reproductive medicine.

New knowledge practices, including new norms, are introduced. Innovation is promoted, and the boundaries of the existing social and political order are transgressed or shifted. The social consequences of ARTs for embryonic personhood, family building and gender are not reflected. Embryos are mostly presented as independent bodies in the transfer from the petri dish into the uterus. Yet incipient forms of unfamiliar relatedness shine through: embryos as quasi-sacred pre-persons and pre-kin. The main focus is the future, with the possibility of a take-home baby and the familiar kinship status of parenthood. A technoscientific rationale with a commercial and spiritual tinge characterises the texts, whereas pictures convey positive feelings through images of happy babies, children and parents, signifying the continuing ideal of the heterosexual nuclear family. This kind of 'embodied progress' (Franklin 1997) is debated here more or less without ethical concern.

ARTs and embryos made by religious experts

Religious institutions have created quite another discourse. Though it is hardly found in newspapers and similar publications, it appears in media communiqués published on the internet. Interesting insights into religious conceptualisations of ARTs, the embryo and kinship are provided by comments on legal drafts, such as one on the popular vote about research with embryonic stem cells in 2004; the comment on the law that should allow preimplantation genetic diagnosis (PDG) in 2005; and the comment on the law on human research in 2006. I analyse here examples of the public discourses of the largest religious groups in Switzerland: Catholics and Protestants.[3]

Catholic embryo tales

The Bioethics Commission (Bioethik-Kommission) of the Swiss Bishops' Conference (SBK) was founded in 2002. What kind of meanings does this religious body create about ARTs and the embryo? In 'The Status of Embryos' written by the SBK in 2003 as a comment on the draft of a law on stem cell research, we find that IVF is strongly negatively assessed. The SBK thinks that because this treatment is only successful in approximately one in three cases, the improvement of 'an unsatisfying technique' is not justified, although it is a heavy burden for 'the couple in question'. The Commission's basic argument is: 'Children are not a product that one can claim, but a gift' (Arbeitsgruppe Bioethik der SBK 27.2.2003). In this paper we also find detailed formulations that show that the embryo is conceptualised as a full person:

> (…) about 16 hours after the beginning of fertilisation, through the unification of the chromosomes the genetic individuality of the new human being is fixed. The further development is specific for human beings and individuals, there are no visible leaps of development any more, and this development goes without interferences from outside (active potentiality of the embryo, in contrast to the passive potentiality of egg cells and semen cells). (…) The embryo does not develop *into* a human being but *as* a human being from the beginning. (Arbeitsgruppe Bioethik der SBK 2003: 2)

This is a plea for the protection of the embryo. For the same reasons, the SBK is inclined to confer basic rights to the embryo when it says:

> the embryo is a potential legal subject. (…) Concerning the right for life the embryo enjoys the same basic rights protection as a person in an uncontested way. (Arbeitsgruppe Bioethik der SBK 2003: 3)

This also applies to so-called 'leftover embryos in vitro'. In the opinion of these experts, scientific knowledge cannot justify research that implies the destruction of embryos to gain stem cells. It is important to note that religious experts, unlike medical experts, make no distinction between a fertilised egg and an embryo. The SBK is also against preimplantation genetic diagnosis (PGD) because they consider it a eugenics policy, arguing that distinguishing acceptable from unacceptable embryos is arbitrary. The following statement shows the core of the SBK's embryo tale – a kin-like relationship of the embryo with God, explicit personhood, implicit sacredness and future potential:

> In the light of Christian faith, human life is a gift of God which has to be protected from the first moment. From conception onwards, every human being is created by God and according to his image and resemblance. A human being has therefore always to be respected as a person. This also applies to the embryo. Finally, it possesses an active potential that it will realise in the properties of an adult person. (SBK 2.12.2005).

Drafts of the constitutional article and law on human research of the same year are particularly criticised firstly because the 'fetus' is not considered a priori as a person but as an 'appendix dependent on its mother'. These drafts are further criticised because only the mother can decide about 'the embryo and the fetus' in case of research on pregnancy. It is argued that fetal surgery is not applied to a 'thing' but to a 'person'. Therefore strict limitations for reusing embryos and fetuses are called for (SBK 29.5.2006). In one of its latest communiqués, a comment on the cultivation of human embryos for therapeutic purposes, the SBK writes that it is against 'designer-babies' and that the human embryo is not a 'replacement deposit' (*Ersatzteillager*). The reason put forward is that 'donor embryos' which do not meet the requirements of the receiver will be 'killed'. Instead, a central registration of living donors for families with sick children is proposed (SBK, 7.6.2006).

Summarising, we can state that reproductive medicine is considered a deficient technique for procreation in the official Catholic view. The embryo as the quintessence of human life and God-likeness has to be protected from its very beginning. In line with this clear-cut and dominant notion of the embryo as a sacred, quasi-autonomous and atomistic person, only a vague notion of kinship and family, of the familiar kind, is expressed in these texts. The relatedness between the embryo and God seems much stronger here than between the embryo and the mother, whose decision-making about the embryo is questioned. With this image of the mother in mind, we cannot only speak of a knowledge practice of normalisation but of retraditionalisation.

Protestant embryo tales

Let us now look at the Protestant discourse, exemplified by the voice of the Swiss Evangelic Church Council (SEK). Only some of their communiqués since 2000 deal with reproductive issues, but they do so in an elementary way, based on theological and ethical considerations. The standpoint of the SEK regarding biotechnologies in general was formulated in a declaration on the popular vote about the law on stem cell research in 2004. Interestingly, biotechnologies, including ARTs, are principally considered positively, in contrast to the Catholic doctrine which assesses these technologies as a failure. Reproductive technologies are included in the endeavour of 'cultivating the earth' and are seen in opposition to nature:

> With assistance of the new biotechnologies, mankind widens its control over nature. This enables mankind to improve the conditions of life and to combat environmental harm. The theological justification for this is found in the command of God to cultivate and to preserve the earth. According to the Christian doctrine, the control of humankind is not unlimited. People have to justify themselves before God, the creator of all things. The SEK places itself in this religious tradition. (SEK 15.10.2004)

Related to the law on research using leftover embryos and embryonic stem cells, the meaning that the Council assigns to the embryo is explicitly expounded in a public statement to the Ministry of Health in 2002 (SEK 29.8.2002). The embryo principally reveals human and 'personal life' (*personales Leben*). Personhood (*Personsein*) according to this theological credo is based on the 'similarity of human beings with God's image' and in the relationship with God and (later on) with people (SEK 2002: 1). Due to the relationship of the embryo with God from its early emergence, it should be respected and treated with protective dignity. The SEK crucially postulates that embryonic personhood is dependent on the 'dialogical character of being human': 'a human being only exists in dependence of Others and towards Others' (2002: 2). This reasoning stresses the perspective of relatedness, including non-human and human kinship. The SBK, in contrast, emphasises the autonomous individual from the very beginning, the pinnacle of enlightenment philosophy, one could argue, and thus de-emphasises relatedness.

A 'leftover embryo' cannot develop into a 'personality' (*Persönlichkeit*). The SEK holds that a zygote, as a 'pile of cells' – in medical terms, synonymous with a fertilised egg – does not stimulate the same emotions as a person in the intensive care unit of a hospital. A crucial categorical difference is further constructed between a person without and a person with personality, which parallels a classification of the embryo versus the fetus. 'Normally', the SEK argues, emotions arise towards personalities who have developed a character and a life history. This kind of personality begins with the interaction of the 'fetus' with other people and its environment. But this agency of the fetus 'is given' only with its nesting in the womb (2002: 3).

The fetus is interestingly represented as an active subject who begins to interact with its environment through its attachment in the motherly body. This active fetus is contrasted with a passive 'leftover embryo', including a zygote. This embryo also has to be considered as a person, but it misses part of its personhood. It will never be able to react to its 'gift of life' because 'socially and objectively mediated relationships with other people' are impossible. It thus becomes an isolated being, 'reduced to itself'. In the following key sentence the different Protestant view from the Catholic on the 'leftover embryo' is impressively stated:

> Even when the leftover embryo *is* a person, it will never *as* a person mature *up to a personality*. (SEK 2002: 3)

Basically, the SEK condemns the purposeful production of embryos that are then destroyed. Therapeutic cloning is also critically considered. Economically, a renunciation of stem cell research would not be a real problem, and Switzerland's status as a research site would not be really damaged. At the same time, the SEK remarks that a clear judgement about the use of 'leftover embryos' is impeded by the idea that they will never develop into personalities with a unique character and life history. Finally, no unequivocal decision is made but strict ethical regulations and the protection of the leftover embryos in favour of the dignity of human life are advocated.

In sum, the Protestant as well as the Catholic discourse on ARTs and the embryo are driven by a religious rationale with a technoscientific tinge. Both show a clear ethical impetus, in contrast to the medical discourse. Unlike Catholic doctrine, in Protestant doctrine, IVF is valued positively and market criteria are also taken into consideration. In both views, the embryo is a sacred autonomous person. But the Protestant reasoning is subtler: more weight is put on the developing embryo as a person with personality. This embryo is an active agent, a full person and relative. It is involved in a kin relation with a decision-making God who makes gifts of life on the one hand, and with a decision-making mother and 'others' on the other. These embryo tales agree, however, on the issue of abortion, but that issue cannot be elaborated upon here.

ARTs and embryos made by mothers

Now I present the views and normalising strategies regarding ARTs and embryos of five mothers who did not experience IVF themselves.[4] I focus on women because they are more bodily and medically involved in relationships with embryos than men. When medical experts normalise ARTs they do so on the base of their medical knowledge, the biological; Christian experts use normalising strategies based on religious or theological ideas, or the sacred. Rana and her sister argue from a lay religious perspective. Rana (29) is married, has one child and belongs to an independent Protestant church. She works part-time as an interior decorator. Her sister (37), a nurse in a gynaecological ward, visited her at the time of the interview and also participated. Rana shows that she is medically informed, when she gives her opinion on ARTs. At first she mentions the treatment with hormones, which she thinks is expensive. Then she says:

> I know that it does not always function the first time, and that it is nerve-racking. But that can also happen if you wait for a child in the natural way. It is always like that if you wish to have a child.

Regarding the restrictiveness of ARTs in Switzerland, she says:

> It's good that you can do something if you cannot get a child, for sure. But there is also a lot of playing, I mean, one just tries. And that is always the case if one interferes. [Restrictions are good] so that human beings cannot play too much as if they were God.

When asked how she defines an embryo or a fetus, Rana gives again evidence of medically informed knowledge: 'At first it is a zygote (*Vorkernstadium*), then an embryo, and when you recognise the limbs it is a fetus.' Her sister interjects: 'Yes, but the question is: When is it life? That is the ethical issue of the whole topic.' Rana thinks that it is life from the first second on, therefore she also rejects research with 'leftover embryos'. At this point the sister intervenes:

> They emerge anyway through IVF. They emerge numerously because they implant about three [embryos] because the probability of success is very small. I think one in ten. (…) Yes I am a nurse and I deal directly with these women. (…) [They] are suffering extremely because it often does not work. (…) Therefore I advocate restriction so that we cannot interfere too much. (…) I see also many disadvantages in medicine in general, many disadvantages: these interferences, this is playing God.

Both sisters view IVF as a technology which is burdensome and which can easily fail. Personhood is attributed to new life from the beginning, and it should not be destroyed. In the last instance they do not refer explicitly to nature, biology or to social relationships of relatedness, but to God. 'Nature' seems to be substituted by 'God', and the embryo is conceptualised as sacred, at least implicitly. They use neither naturalising nor socialising strategies (Thompson 2005). Their rhetoric strategies resemble the Catholic discourse, although they are Protestant.

The rhetoric of Ines, a former midwife, has also sacred features. Ines (27) is married and has one child. She got pregnant unexpectedly and initially did not intend to live with the father of the child. Like Rana and her sister, Ines is ambivalent about the desire to have a child with ARTs. She thinks that it gives too much scope to family forms other than the heterosexual nuclear one. In particular, she is sceptical about sonography and prenatal tests because her doctor made a wrong diagnosis, and she comments: 'That little baby is still so protected in the belly and also has the right not yet to be delivered to the world.'

Ines feels close to nature. Related to the use of 'leftover embryos' for research she remarks:

> Yes, I am just a natural woman. (…) If you would ask me: You have a strongly disabled child in your belly and it is only in the tenth week of pregnancy, but I know that it cannot survive. I would not conduct abortion. (…) One should leave it with the parents who want the eggs for their child, and afterwards one should not go on and use them for other purposes. (…) I would find it better if we would research more on how we can preserve nature, or something like that.

Ines' identity as a 'natural woman' is inspired by a Buddhist-like spiritualism. This is the frame of her ideas on ARTs and the embryo:

> I think life does not stop and does not begin. (…) I am not a Buddhist but I have a kind of Buddhist conception that we have a consciousness or a spirit, or how could you call it, who continues to exist, before and after birth. (…) I just believe in reincarnation. (…) It has nothing to do with religion, or such things.

Partnership and family are not explicit issues in this interview. The embryo is implicitly represented as a dependent kinship entity and is hardly geneticised. Motherhood, 'the child', its rights and its protection, as well as a Bhuddist-like cosmology about nature, are the foci of Ines' narrative. Her conception of the sacred is not associated with God but with a spiritualised conception of the natural. This conception of the natural is of another character than the biological in the sense of biogenetic substance.

Next, we turn to two mothers who confer sacredness, personhood, and kin qualities upon the embryo and its development into a future child. They all abhor research on embryos and their commodification. For all of them, adoption would be a better alternative than burdensome treatments with ARTs. They reject the social effects of ARTs because of moral criteria. Subsequently, all of them support the existing kinship and gender order, particularly the currently existing heterosexual nuclear family and its specific kind of motherhood.

Instead of spiritual substance, Julia (32) stresses biogenetic substance related to one's 'own child'. She lives in a domestic partnership and has one child. As an architect, she is fascinated by these technologies. Regarding ARTs and embryos, she can imagine making use of a surrogate mother, but only a morally sound one, and only if she were also guaranteed to receive the child back. She also would donate 'leftover embryos' for research. Concerning visualising and monitoring technologies she is ambivalent, though due to the experience of pregnancy loss. And only in this context she uses the term 'embryo':

> My body had not noticed it. They had seen it on the ultra sound. And then he [the doctor] said: either I could have it taken out or take a pill and then wait until the body notices it. And then I thought: no, no, it should immediately be taken out. I don't want to carry a dead embryo in me.

She talks about her situation as a 'super risky pregnancy' because her doctors saw on the ultra sound image that she was carrying one-egg-twins, but categorised the embryos as genetically defective. Julia interestingly comments: 'Losing the pregnancy actually meant something was genetically wrong. And that strongly calmed me down.'

Julia uses genetic knowledge to normalise the critical situation of pregnancy loss and the wish for a child with her own biogenetic substance. In this context she conceptualises the 'embryo' as an entity between life and death. And in the case of definite death, she cannot wait to get rid of it. During her successful pregnancy she conceptualised the beginning of life as a 'child', and thus constructed kinship rather with the fetus and during a later phase of pregnancy than with the embryo in the early phase. Julia explicitly argues in a biological way, on the one hand to normalise procreation with ARTs, and on the other hand, in favour of technical and social innovations. Her rhetorical strategy comes closest to those in medical discourse. Subsequently, we also find here a tension between geneticised conservatism and social innovation.

Nadja (41) was educated as a teacher and works as a press spokeswoman. Like Julia, she lives in a domestic partnership, has one child, and also experienced a pregnancy loss. Regarding ARTs and related research she takes a less rational stance and is more ambivalent than Julia, but she has no moral objections. She supports, for example, donor insemination for singles and lesbian women, but she rejects surrogacy because of possible commercialisation and because she thinks that a mother has a strong relationship with 'the child'. Asked what an embryo is, she immediately tells about her earlier pregnancy loss:

> You have certain feelings. I have experienced that with the pregnancy that did not continue. It was after eight weeks. It was still so tiny that it was hardly visible. You hardly can see it with your eyes. And nevertheless you are sad as if it concerns a living human being, if you experience it yourself. Otherwise I would say: A fertilised egg, what is that anyway? (…) It is a personal value. If it is from Walter [her partner] and me, I have another relationship towards it.

She thus thinks that after eight weeks an embryo is not yet a person, but something personal and a sign of partnership. Like Julia, she uses the term 'it' and 'child' for the beginning of life, and she uses 'embryo' only in the context of her pregnancy loss, and thus of death:

> (…) I had to go to the hospital at that time to scratch out the embryo, a horrible word, but it is like that. And I don't know after all what they did with it. But I have said goodbye before. It did not mean anything for me any more, and it was also not alive.

During the first three months of her second pregnancy she was eager to undergo several tests, sonography and also chorion biopsy, to check whether the child had genetic defects as her pregnancy was evaluated as risky because of her age. When the test results came back indicating a healthy pregnancy, she used to show the ultrasound pictures around at any occasion. Nadja is a mother for whom the social is most important. She does not conceptualise relatedness with the embryo based on biogenetic imagination, at least not explicitly, but mainly based on notions of the particular sociality of partnership. Her strategy of socialisation is also more related to innovation, technically and socially, than to preserving the existing social order. Her rhetoric contests both medical and religious discourse.

In short, the first three women value ARTs and related research rather negatively, the fourth is ambivalent and the fifth has a positive attitude. Based on different beliefs, or cosmologies, and biographical experience, these mothers construct the embryo surprisingly differently. They conceive the embryo as a full person and relative, as women often seem to do today. As spiritually minded mothers they also strongly sacralise it. The women who experienced pregnancy loss consider the embryo in different ways as a pre-person and pre-relative, an entity between life and death.

Conclusions

These 'embryo tales' contain important elements of Swiss conception or origin stories (Yanagisako and Delaney 1995). They show a broad range of contested meanings about ARTs and the embryo, and at the same time they reflect basic understandings and priorities regarding kinship, the social order and cosmology (Franklin 1999). Embryos made in Switzerland are surprising persons and relatives: with full, semi, potential or possibly-becoming status. This makes their investigation scientifically relevant. It is also politically relevant because of the impact these understandings have on ethical debates during law making and on social assessments of current and future biomedical practices. This analysis shows that embryos are often, but not always, conceptualised as autonomous persons and kin entities. If the embryo is conceived of as kin, a whole range of rhetorical strategies are used to mark that. But can we always speak of a mixture of naturalisation and socialisation strategies in the way Thompson (2005) suggests? The mothers, who identify themselves as religious, seem to defy this suggestion. The spiritual rhetoric can hardly be understood with her model (see also de Jong, this volume).

Based on David Schneider's (1986) research, Thompson assumes that for Euro-Americans, kinship is first and foremost based on biogenetic substance. Although she deals with the sacredness of the embryo, she neither reflects on its kin properties, nor upon the issue of normalisation in a spiritual or religious context. I think we should argue more subtly. This study shows that women with a strong spiritual or religious orientations negotiate their meanings about procreation, the embryo and kinship in the context of ARTs mainly related to spiritual substance, as religious experts do. In their rhetoric on reproduction, biogenetic substance is for a large part replaced by spiritual substance. Therefore, I propose to expand Thompson's model, so that a strategy that conceives biogenetic substance as spiritual, or nature as spiritual, can be classified as a socialising strategy as well. This research reveals knowledge practices about the embryo that are no doubt informed by biomedical thinking. But in the last instance, normalisation in all the embryo tales is achieved through legitimising strategies based in different ways on the sacred, the natural, the biological and the social.

The newness of ARTs is not only normalised in a retraditionalised way in the cases presented, but ARTs are also considered as a further chance for technical and social innovation, as in Thompson's study. The Protestant conceptualisation of the embryo as a person without personality enables a conservative or an innovative kin relationship between mother and future child and their social context, unlike the Catholic one. The socialising strategies of Protestant kinship making, based on sacred and social arguments, have the potential to contest the existing conditions of kinship, the social order and cosmology. The embryo as a sacred pre-kin person, 'a person without personality' but in close relationship with God, seems to be dwelling in a liminal space between life and death, not only physically but also socially – and in the interstices between retraditionalisation and innovation. However, the secular women, who in these cases experienced pregnancy loss, do not conceive the embryo as a person but as a pre-person and pre-kin entity, lingering in a semi-social space between life and death. They relate to it either by naturalising or by socialising strategies of normalisation that are explicitly innovative.

Notes

[1] This interview material has been collected in cooperation with students of a university course in anthropology on the body and technologies. The course included an explorative study on the imagined effects of ARTs on kinship, gender and the body (de Jong et al. 2007). Interviews were conducted in German. Of the sixteen interviewees, twelve were women. I thank the students for their collaboration and informants for the permission to use their data.

[2] Bundesamt für Statistik 2007. Statistik der medizinisch unterstützten Fortpflanzung. Behandlungszyklen 2006. Neuchâtel.

[3] In 2000 41.8% of the population were members of the Catholic church, 33.0% of the Protestant church, albeit not all practising members. Further, 1.8% of the population belong to small Christian communities, including Orthodox Christians, and 4.3% are Muslims (Schuler et al. 2007: 128).

[4] For a quantitative study on attitudes of Swiss IVF parents on 'surplus embryos' (sic) see Mohler-Kuo et al. 2009.

References

Bock v. Wülfingen, B. (2006) Love and health in the geneticisation of conception: a discourse analysis exploring the transformation of imaginative spaces, Unpublished Paper.

de Jong, W., Ashgedom, Ph., Egger, S.V., Isabaeva, E., Karmova, B., Mader, M., Menn, J., Pfenninger, N., Rinderknecht, A. and Vollenweider, I. (2007) Reproduktionstechnologien zwischen Neuerfindung und Traditionalisierung von Körper, Verwandtschaft und Geschlecht in der deutschen Schweiz. Eine ethnologische Pilotstudie, Unveröffentlichter Bericht. Zürich: Ethnologisches Seminar.

Edwards, J. ([1993] 1999) Explicit connections: ethnographic inquiry in North-West England, in J. Edwards, S. Franklin, E. Hirsch, F. Pine and M. Strathern *Technologies of Procreation: Kinship in the Age of Assisted Conception*. London, New York: Routledge: 60-90.

Franklin, S. (1997) *Embodied Progress: A Cultural Account of Assisted Conception*, London, New York: Routledge.

Franklin, S. ([1993] 1999). Making representations: the parliamentary debate on the human fertilisation and embryology act, in J. Edwards, S. Franklin, E. Hirsch, F. Pine and M. Strathern *Technologies of Procreation. Kinship in the Age of Assisted Conception*, London, New York: Routledge: 127-165.

Franklin, S. (2006) The IVF-stem cell interface, *International Journal of Surgery*, 4: 86-90.

Hirsch, E. ([1993] 1999) Negotiated limits: interviews in South-East England, in J. Edwards, S. Franklin, E. Hirsch, F. Pine and M. Strathern *Technologies of Procreation: Kinship in the Age of Assisted Conception*, London, New York: Routledge: 91-121.

Kaufman, S.R. and Morgan, L.M. (2005) The anthropology of the beginnings and ends of life, *Annual Review of Anthropology* 34: 317-341.

Mohler-Kuo, M., Zellweger, U. Duran, A., Hohl, M.K, Gutzwiler, F. and M. Mutsch (2009) Attitudes of couples towards the destination of surplus embryos, *Human Reproduction*, 1(1): 1-9.

Morgan, L. 2003. Embryo tales, in S. Franklin and M. Lock (eds) *Remaking Life and Death: Toward an Anthropology of the Biosciences*. Santa Fe, New Mexico: School of American Research Press: 261-292.

Schneider, D.M. (1986) *American Kinship: A Cultural Account*, Chicago, London: University of Chicago Press.

Schuler, M., Dessemontet, P., Jemelin, C., Jarne, A., Pasche, N. und Haug, W. (2007) *Atlas des räumlichen Wandels der Schweiz / Atlas des mutations spatiales de la Suisse*. Bundesamt für Statistik, Zürich: Verlag Neue Zürcher Zeitung.

Strathern, M. (2005) *Kinship, Law and the Unexpected: Relatives Are Always a Surprise*. Cambridge: Cambrige University Press.

Thompson, C. (2005) *Making Parents: The Ontological Choreography of Reproductive Technologies*. Cambridge MA, London: MIT Press.

Yanagisako, S. and Delaney, C. (1995) Naturalizing power, in S. Yanagisako and C. Delaney (eds) *Naturalizing Power: Essays in Feminist Cultural Analysis*. London, New York: Routledge: 1-22.

'Ersatz children' in the Russian media: reproductive technologies and cyborgisation

Olga Brednikova

In one of the most widespread Russian newspapers *Argumenty i Fakty*, Arguments and Facts, the reasons for turning to reproductive technologies and in vitro fertilisation are described as follows:

> According to statistics, one in four married couples in Russia cannot have children in a natural way. So they are left with an 'unnatural' way – in vitro fertilisation (IVF). For this purpose, an ovum is taken from a woman, a sperm cell is 'forcedly' integrated into it in vitro, a tiny embryo is grown in the incubator for several days and then it is sent 'to its addressee' – that is, a woman's womb, where the whole process was meant to have taken place without medical interference. I have seen the incubator where new young people are 'collected': it is very humid inside, the temperature is strictly kept at 37°, though it looks like an ordinary fridge. The difference is that the ordinary fridge contains sausages and yesterday's chicken broth, while this one contains vials where a cell binds to a cell, new LIFE emerges, a PERSON appears. (AiF 13.04.2005)

This extract allows us to see the complex and ambiguous attitude prevailing in Russia related to assisted reproduction technologies (ARTs), and to decipher the numerous meanings that are attributed to them. For example, the text renders the queer and abnormal nature of the procedure in its descriptions: 'is 'forcedly' integrated' and 'unnatural way'. It also shows the perception of infertility as a problem, an appalling beginning of technologisation. It further displays the mysterious and at the same time 'down-to-earth' nature of science as it becomes everyday knowledge, for example 'the incubator where new young people are 'collected'' is compared to 'an ordinary fridge with sausages and broth'. But I was mostly attracted by the last sentence about growing a person: 'a cell binds to a cell'. Moreover, it is not just a phrase about 'a person's' growing but 'a PERSON'S' growing, creating a special status for the child. One of the central characters of the media narrations about ARTs is the child that appears with the help of these technologies. In this essay I ask how are ART children problematised and, consequently, how are they constituted in media discourse. I am also interested in the production of their subjectivity, and how their 'difference' is constituted. By this I mean how their 'otherness' and the novelty of these new subjects and subjectivities are included into the existing social order or, conversely, transform it.

The study materials are newspaper publications between 1996 and 2006 dealing with ARTs, specifically personal stories, governmental policies and advertisements for clinics that practice these technologies. Two newspapers were chosen for the analysis: *Rossiyskaya Gazeta* (RG), the Russian Newspaper, an official governmental publication; and *Argumenty I Fakty* (AiF), Arguments and Facts, the most widespread popular, or yellow press, newspaper in Russia. The choice of these newspapers was determined by an assumption that these two publications represent and interpret ARTs differently, creating different meanings of these news technologies; but this research has shown that there are no major differences between them. Both newspapers problematise ARTs similarly, they use the same interpretive schemes, vocabularies, and they even provide comments from the same experts. For this discourse analysis two methods were used: social categorisation analysis and conceptual analysis (Silverman 1995).

'Ersatz Children'

The newspaper article quoted at the beginning of this essay tells quite a dramatic story of a woman who was trying to become a mother for many years. After a long period of infertility treatment and numerous attempts with IVF, she finally succeeded in becoming a mother of twins who were carried by a surrogate mother. The last sentence in this happily ending story is: 'Her children do not even have a clue that they are 'ersatz'' (AiF 13.04.2005). Children born as a result of ARTs are called 'ersatz' here. The use of quotation marks demonstrates a certain conventionalism of the definition. At the same time, such a signification draws a boundary, detaching ART children from other children, the so-called 'real' children. Newspapers publications use numerous designations for ART children. 'In vitro children' is the most widespread name, but 'immaculate conception children' (RG 15.02.2002), 'born in secrecy' (RG 21.02.2006), and even 'clone children' (RG 27.09.2002) – though the article describes IVF and not cloning – are also used. Certainly, such denominations represent their 'otherness'.

Such children are watched closely, they are constantly evaluated. Their otherness is produced and fixed by endless comparisons with children born without technological use. In this case we observe, in my opinion, a post-modern self-constitution through mirroring the other:

> They differ in absolutely no way from those who came into this world in a traditional way. They are children like others. And only their parents and doctors know the secret of their birth (…). (RG 06.08.1998)

An attempt is made to equalise all children, but at the same time an image of ART children is created in which they are portrayed as better quality children, both physically and socially. In this way, ART children are classified as a special group, while this peculiar positioning solidifies the boundary. Below I am going to analyse their 'otherness' with respect to Haraway's (2005) concept of the cyborg, the creation of early subjectivities and damaged social identities.

Cyborg children

The technology of linking female and male germ cells during IVF is described in the newspaper publications in great detail and in a very lively style. Readers are given a description of each phase, step-by-step. All the 'mysteries' of technological 'child production' are unveiled:

> This surgery differs from those in ordinary hospitals. (…) There is no admittance of unauthorised personnel to this room. And this is also right: a mystery is a mystery. It is created by specialists of invitro fertilisation in the Moscow Centre for Family the Planning and Reproduction of Human beings. An ovum is taken from a woman in a surgery, and then it is placed into a special medium and given to the laboratory through the special window. It takes the ovum three to four hours to adapt to the new environment. If it goes fine – and it is watched under a microscope – sperm cells are added to this medium. An embryo in a small transparent glass – it is called a Petri dish – is placed into an incubator that looks like an ordinary fridge. (RG 09.01.1998)

It is important to note that the language used to describe these procedures is not medical, but rather technological. Assisted reproductive technologies are practiced in medical institutions, but these are presented in print media as scientific laboratories rather than as a therapeutic clinical setting. This discourse obviously constitutes these technologies not as medical procedures aimed at infertility treatment, but as technical manipulations aimed at 'child creation'.

The technological vocabulary of medical engineering practically eliminates human passions and suffering. It rather mystifies us and invites us into science fiction, or even into an exciting game with the goal of the creation of a new person. The metaphor of the game was created and elaborated by members of a feminist artists group called *subRosa*, and their fiction correlates and interlaces with the newspapers' fiction:

> Any woman exposed to reproductive technologies simultaneously becomes the main character and focus of an intense drama, which is comparable to a multi-layered video game, taking part in a series of carefully planned actions that more often end up with a tragedy rather than a victory. The game plot is an amazingly rationalised creation of life. The sequence of actions demonstrates heroic colonial conquest of steady (infertile) bodies and genes by fertility doctors. (…). An embryo is a trophy regained from the Dark Continent by the Deus ex molecular biology machina. (subRosa 2004: 2)

In my opinion this text is quite compatible with the previous quotation describing the 'mysterious' technology and with the following phrase:

> Just imagine what kind of devices, instruments and specimens are required for this process! How fine the mastery of medics! Unconsciously a feeling of fantasy and mystics appears (RG 09.01.1998).

Thus, ART children are constituted as products of almost fantastic medical engineering and have nothing to do with feelings and intimacy. They are the products of an immaculate conception, as these technologies are called in the newspaper article (RG 20.08.1999). The technologisation of child production transforms children into cyborgs. As a result of ARTs, they become a complex combination, a constellation of technology and human body, like Haraway's (2005: 323-324) description of the cyborg:

> (…) a cross-breed of a machine and an organism, a creation of social reality and at the same time an invention of fiction.

From this perspective, the boundary between technology and human beings becomes 'blurred and unclear' (Thacker 2004: 8). In Russian public discourse, a cyborg child is constituted first of all as an achievement of scientific technological progress, but also as a 'scientific nature assistant'. At the same time, a cyborg child becomes the object of uncertain, inarticulate fears or, following Michael Mulkay (1996: 157), the object of fears of 'Frankenstein archetypes'. These fears are manifested in the separation and segregation of 'cyborg children' as well as in the production of their 'otherness' that is not only technological but also and even more social.

ART children's early subjectivity

The 'otherness' of children conceived through the use of ARTs starts long before their birth. It is quite evident that because of the development of medical technologies, the embryo's ambivalent status as a subject, whose 'personality is immanent but not eminent' (Conclin and Morgan 1996: 658), has become more obvious. An embryo has come to be perceived as a person, even though one that is not yet revealed. According to Conklin and Morgan (1996: 658), the way people in Western cultures try to overcome and resolve the ambivalent position of embryos can be considered as 'the involvement of body models that localize personality in specific body characteristics'. These authors argue that the bodily incarnation of an embryo allows its perception as a person. New medical technologies of visualisation, ultra-sound examinations in particular, enable us to see the body of future children, which definitely stimulates and activates the production of embryonic subjectivity. The most vivid evidence of this, which I show elsewhere, is the creation of a documented individual life story by putting the ultra-sound examination printout into a family or personal photo album (Brednikova 2008). Thus, the embryo, perceived as a subject, comes under influence and control of special structures. For example, in contemporary Russia, prenatal pedagogy and prenatal psychology are being developed and institutionalised. These new disciplines are focused on, and consequently control, the upbringing, education and health of an unborn and unrevealed child.

ARTs broaden the limits of such subjectivity by redefining the borderline between nature and human beings. Having introduced autonomous conception into common practice, medicine takes an active part in the production of similarly autonomous subjects, separated from the mother's body. Physicians literally 'make' a new person in vitro and then place her into the mother's body just for a period of nine months, after which she will regain autonomy. Special knowledge about embryonic development enables medicine to correct and treat an unborn person. Thus, ARTs allow the constitution of an ovum as a subject even prior to its implantation into a mother's body. This is visible in Russian ART debates. Certainly, embryos are not yet perceived as full-bodied subjects; but these debates make room for these perspectives and show promise for such developments in the future. In particular, ARTs have initiated a discussion of the legal status of an ovum regarding property rights and responsibilities and also regarding the fundamental rights of any person – the right to life. It is interesting to note that this debate exists separately from both abortion debates and debates in embryonic studies in which the status of embryos is also quite problematic. In Russian public debates today, the issue of abortion has gradually become less controversial, while publications on this topic are less frequent (Zdravomyslova 2009). However, discussions aboutu embryonic studies, in which embryos are considered valuable study material (Mickley 1994, 1996; Kirejczyk 2008), hardly exist in Russia because embryology is not yet developed.

Thanks to the popularisation of medical knowledge about fertilisation and embryonic development for parents using ARTs, a child starts already with ova and sperm discharge and their interconnection. The personalisation of a prospective child begins in the private family sphere, and it begins with naming. With ARTs, a conception is not an accident but an accomplishment within a specific life project. Prospective parents invent names and give them to their children during 'the production process':

> The first and second time when it did not work out, as the embryos would not 'stick', I was not even upset. There was no one to bewail. But the third time it started working, my and my husband's cells successfully united and two embryos at once were implanted into me: An'ka and Van'ka. We called them so immediately. (AiF 13.04.2005)

By naming a prospective person, that person is already transformed into a certain personality. We cannot say that giving a name to a not-yet-implanted ovum is a normalised and widespread practice but this tendency already exists. In online forums, women undergoing ART treatment discuss their frozen embryos and give them tender nicknames, calling them snowflakes, snow-queens or kings. Frozen embryos with nicknames are 'not-quite people', not yet personalities with concrete names. Active attempts to make the process of using ARTs less technological and more humane are needed to create conditions for, and to redefine the limits of the natural and the social, as well as the production of new and early subjectivities.

Besides personalisation, giving the embryo social identities also produces early subjectivity. According to media publications, the 'products' of ARTs already possess social identities, primarily ethnic identities that are often related to religious identities. Moreover, identities are perceived as essentials passed from genetic parents to children. How social identification is inscribed upon prospective children is not described obviously, it is rather problematised in publications on genetic relationships and becomes most evident in articles on male reproductive donorship:

> Already, sperm donors with different blood groups and of different nationalities are required. The clinic database only contains one donor with negative rhesus factor and only one Muslim. (RG 16.12.2003)

Among different personal and social characteristics the ethnic identity of the donors is mostly problematised because its inheritance admits no doubts:[1]

> Notwithstanding the detailed donor description, you are playing a lottery. First of all, the questionnaire does not provide information on bloods mixed in potential fathers. Even if he is Russian, his mother could well be half-Georgian and his grandfather, a Tatar. Moreover a donor's features could come up in several generations. And then you get a grandson looking like his distant ancestor and you should explain to everybody that you didn't succeed in guessing the questionnaire's data. (AiF 15.06.2004)

Thus, a sperm cell united with an ovum in vitro imbues the prospective child with social identities. Moreover, an ova which is not yet implanted into a woman's body is already perceived as a personality with its own name and personal history, it receives a biography. The analysis so far shows that we can talk of an early subjectivity of ART children. Perhaps this early embryo subjectivity can be interpreted as an attempt to make a cyborg more human and to overcome its technological nature. These definitions and descriptions of differences specify ART children in a certain way and produces their 'otherness'.

ART children in search for their 'identity'

ART children's otherness, which so far has been defined by the peculiar way of their conception, is further actively produced through their unclear and uncertain identity. As Donna Haraway wrote, cyborgs have a deficient and crashed social identity (Haraway 1991: 331). This is also represented in the newspaper articles:

> The greatest scientific achievement conceived pro bono of the humanity turned out to be a tragedy for many people. (…) First, in vitro children grew up and some of them started looking for their biologic fathers, or, scientifically said, for their identity. (RG 27.09.2002)

According to these publications, children conceived through sperm donorship sooner or later feel their otherness. Trying to solve the mystery of their birth, such children question who their 'real' father is and make attempts to find him. Interestingly, there are no publications about IVF children looking for their 'real mother'. To demonstrate the dramatic nature of the situation, I quote part of a newspaper article dedicated to discussion of such children in the Western world, though there are also such publications about the Russian context:

> Rebecca cannot stop searching. Something inside her desires to learn who she is, after all. 'Who am I, where did I come from and where am I going? (…) He is part of my life and I wanted to know who I am'. (RG 27.09.2002)

This emotional quotation demonstrates the depth of this person's tragedy. But if we leave emotional responses in brackets, it is possible to reconstruct a suggestive identification matrix constituting social relationships and normative social order. We see then that the reasons for Rebecca's identity crisis are connected primarily to uncertainty about her origins. Interestingly, 'mystery' is one of the most widespread categories used for the description of reproductive donorship.

The production of self or personality occurs through seeking genetic relationships. But this search for genetic origins is not connected to uncovering a real father or a new family. Knowledge about genetic parents becomes sacral knowledge through which ART children finally discover their identity. There are two fatherly references for ART children: the social and the genetic father. With respect to the former, social differences are more important and social distance is created; but in relation to the latter, intimacy develops because of physical similarity because there is no social history of the relationship:

> Bill claims that even though he did not know anything, he suspected something since his childhood. 'My father and I, we were completely different. He was small and well-muscled with acrid tough manners. In contrast to him I was tall, thin and interested in 'unmanly' things like aesthetics and design. He was always alien to me and now I suddenly understood why.' (RG 27.09.2002)

Identity is thus primarily build on the basis of genetic relationship. In both these situations, the social – socialisation and upbringing, social parents and social environment – was not enough, as it did not create an integral, uncontroversial identity. Social experience of being a child of certain parents should be combined primarily to being their genetic child. If social and genetic parenthood are torn it endangers integrity and leads to an identity crisis, or 'broken lives'. A possible solution available is to strictly observe the anonymity of conception. Thus it is strongly advised to choose donors on the basis of ethnic or physical similarity. In summary, the status of genetic history in modern Russian society is extremely important. Subjects are produced only with their revealed genetic history. Individual genetic history is the basis, the source and starting point of personality construction; it is a matrix of social history that is built on a genetic basis.

ART children as a component of a genetic chain

The emergence and the spread of ARTs problematises and disrupts the established social order in many ways. One of these disturbances, according to newspaper publications, is the imputed normal age for a woman to give birth to a child. Violation of age norms creates irony first of all, and is described as a ridiculous comic situation or with amused curiosity:

> A 69-year-old Mexican woman made up her mind to undertake an audacious action. Irma Serrano is an ex-actress and a senator. In her, let's have it straight, considerable age, this lady got pregnant. (…) Irma says she never wanted to have children, then suddenly late in her life this desire came to her and became so intense that she had to turn to doctors for help. (RG 16.12.2003)

Only a complicated situation or a life tragedy legitimises crossing the age borderline. Giving birth to a child when you are 'older than …' is acceptable and fair only if your whole previous life was dedicated to fighting and overcoming infertility. In these cases certain newspaper articles build the biography of a woman as a sequence of steps on the road to motherhood.

Another violation of the social order by ARTs is the disruption of logic and harmony of family relations, a troubling of the dominant concept of a family which is replicated in the mass media:

> Everything is mixed up in Olga T.'s family. Olga is 48. This is her second marriage. Olga's husband is much younger, than she. They both want a baby. But the mother's age is an obstacle. (…) A donor's cell was needed. Olga brought her 20-year-old daughter, who agreed to be the donor, to the Centre for Family Planning and Human Reproduction. The process of artificial insemination passed successfully. Now Olga is pregnant. But how will the family manage to identify kinship relations: who is the mother, who is the sister of this baby? Maybe it doesn't matter? The most important thing is that a child was born. (RG 09.01.1998)

The problem of unclear family relations and statuses is resolved by the importance of the goal: 'a child was born'. The reconstruction of the broken social order, such as reproductive age, the linear and logical nature of family relations, is not at all performed by re-definition of social norms themselves. The main objective of ARTs is the production of children. Childlessness, perceived as a 'malfunction' of the family concept, turns out to be an important violation of the social order. The appearance of a child normalises the situation, reconstructs the standard concept of a family as a chain of generations, and removes any related violation. In media debates on ARTs, these children are given a special role. Their mission is to be a descendant or an inheritor. Interestingly, an inheritor is one of the most common terms for ART children in the print media. Its closest competitor is the term 'in vitro child'.

In 2006 the story of a child born in Russia from a father who died several years ago was extensively discussed in the media. The grandmother of this child took the sperm of her son from a clinic in Israel, where her son was treated, and brought it to Russia, where a child was born with the help of a donated ovum and a surrogate mother. This story generated much public interest. Many publications and TV commentaries covered it and the grandmother appeared in many talk shows. That child does not have either a genetic mother or a genetic father by his side. In fact, at the very moment of his creation, he was a future orphan. After several bureaucratic collisions, his grandmother was formally indicated as a fostering mother on the child's registration documents. But in public, the grandmother still presents herself as a grandmother, not as a mother. From his father, the child inherited the family name and a patronymic, but there is a blank space in the line for the father in his birth certificate. The child is born in a family vacuum. He has no genetic parents and no social ones. He ended up in a gap between the past and the future. Interestingly, the will of living parents to keep the family succession was not involved here, but the logic of genetic continuity is still kept, whether the parents are alive or not.

This story enables us in my opinion to reconstruct the place of a child in the modern social order. The production of a child's subjectivity is performed primarily through his definition as a genetic inheritor. A child is interpreted not as a social inheritor, not as a result of upbringing or socialisation, and not as an inheritor of social status and capital. He is a component of a genetic continuity, the borders of which are defined by the family.

Assisted reproduction helps to overcome infertility problems of genetic continuity on the one hand, but on the other, these technologies also create such problems. Any type of reproductive donation both reconstructs the succession of generations and at the same time makes its genetic basis problematic. Involvement of sperm and ova donors in the fertilisation procedure and the carrying of a child disrupt the 'harmony' and clarity of genetic inheritance. But, as this analysis shows, such a connection is crucial not for both parents, but solely for the prospective father. The genetic relation between a mother and a child is not problematised, and hardly covered. If a donated ovum is used, motherhood is constituted through the nine-month period of carrying the child. If a surrogate mother is used, the identity of the genetic mother is 'self-evident'. When donated sperm is used, the relation between a social father and a child becomes a topic for discussion. It is perceived not only as a problem for the child, as in the examples of identity crisis above, but also for the father. The role of 're-translator of genetic material' is delegated to the father, while a child is defined and perceived as a 'genetic inheritor'.

ART children as 'genetic lego'?

So what does a prospective child inherit from its genetic parents, or in case of donorship, from a donor?

> The questionnaire responses of a [sperm] donor are in front of me: 178 cm tall; born in 1978; Russian; weight, 70 kg; dark blond straight hair; brown eyes; curved nose; oval face. Interests: drawing, music. Education: higher economics. No bad habits.' (AiF 15.06.2004)

In the quotation above, physical and social characteristics of a sperm donor are mixed together, which means that they are equivalent in this context. According to such newspaper articles, knowledge about a donor's personality is important, and not only to enable the prospective parents to choose a reliable and responsible person to build-up a certain relationship. His social characteristics are even more crucial for the prospective child, as it is supposed that the child might inherit them. With the genes not only physical features or liability to certain diseases are inherited, but social identities as well, along with some personal characteristics:

> Attraction to extreme behaviour is also of a genetic nature and can be inherited. Yearning for adventure is inherited as well as eye or hair colour. (AiF 23.4.2003)

According to a current popularised version of genetic research, the social has an extensive genetic basis and genes are assigned a role of re-translating the social. In these public debates, the status of genes is extremely important. Following the anthropologist Rayna Rapp (1991: 384) we can explain this as follows:

> (…) genetics provides metaphors of human perfectability and definitions of the individual as holding within itself own potentialities.

The perception of a genetic determination of the social, replicated in the Russian print media, brings forth the idea that ARTs genetically enable the construction of children, produced on a by-order basis, taking into account parents' wishes. In particular, newspapers vividly discuss the sperm of celebrities, Nobel-prize winners and models and the creation of subsequent ova banks, so that anybody can construct a child according to his or her wishes, planning not only the child's appearance, but also personal and social characteristics. Thus, the presumption that ARTs can genetically design social characteristics of prospective children constitutes ART children as a genetic puzzle with perfect personal characteristics and desired social ones as its elements. But only single women can enjoy a certain freedom and a legitimate right to creatively construct a prospective child. The choice of a donor by married couples is motivated in another way:

> They usually try to find a donor anthropologically similar to the sterile father. The requests of unmarried women are also taken into consideration. They have the right to 'order', for example, European, Caucasian, or Mongoloid race. (AiF 03.02.1999)

Despite the possibilities and perspectives of 'genetic design', it only allows creating an exterior copy to attain outward similarity with the prospective social father. Through this external similarity, the broken genetic continuity is masked, and the broken concept of the family is reconstructed. In print media discourse, ART children are not presented as genetic lego, which would probably not only assert their otherness, but also constitute a kind of superiority. Nowadays they are included into the existing social order and called upon to sustain it, which confirms Mulkay's remark (1994b: 699) regarding debates about ARTs and embryo studies:

> The global effect of public debate (...) is to assure social practices sustaining the conservative idea of a normal family life.

Thus, media debate does not support the radical social potential of ARTs but protects existing norms.

Discursive strategies of normalisation of novelty

In Russian public debates, ARTs remain quite controversial, as often happens with many new technologies. In the 1990s, these technologies were identified with 'far away' places, like the United Kingdom or Mexico, and such cases were presented as ironic curiosities. Later, the reality of ARTs caused certain fears. These fears relate to the disruption of the existing social order, in particular, violation of linear kinship. Today these dangerous novelties are gradually becoming normalised, and ARTs are being slowly incorporated into the existing social order which they are even called upon to protect. At the beginning, the only discursive strategy of normalisation suggested in the media was a strategy of masking or hiding. After that, mystery and secrecy were the most popular categories which discursively constituted ARTs. Authors of newspaper articles write not so much about the mystery of a child's conception, but rather of the mystery of the procedure itself. Gradually, this mystery is transformed into a secret. Donation of reproductive biomaterials is particularly scrupulously protected and disguised. Publications say much about issues such as donor anonymity and ways to keep the secrecy of a child's birth. Such secrecy is in fact simulated responsibility, as it does not solve the problems but rather defers and accumulates them. Perhaps debates about whether secrecy is necessary for couples using ARTs, and especially reproductive donation of eggs and sperm, will not be so important in the future.

In my opinion, the 'enlightenment' stage – a period in which publications disclose in great detail the purpose and content of these technologies – is coming to an end. Now public debate is increasingly oriented toward two discursive strategies of ART normalisation. The first of these is the inclusion of ARTs into public discourses around demographic problems in Russia. In this case, normalisation takes place on the level of national ideology and politics. Thus, numerous publications of recent years actively support the idea of using statistics and expertise. As a rule, the opinion of reproductive scientists and medical officers is that ARTs are a national blessing for Russia as there is a perception that there are not enough children being born.

The second discursive strategy of normalisation takes place on another level. Newspaper articles turn more and more to quasi-private life stories. In almost every publication, 'real' family stories of childless couples, not of single persons, are now told. These couples achieve the happiness of parenthood after long, painful treatment and long-term financial deprivations and suffering. Following Carolyn Michelle (2007: 644), we can say that the meaning and effect of these anecdotal personalisations is to create interest and make 'high-tech' procedures and technologies more relevant and personally meaningful to lay audiences by demonstrating their value for particular individuals.

By turning to 'real life', the technologies are included into 'the real life' and become in fact reality. I consider as most important that in these anecdotal family stories ARTs are primarily normalised through suffering. These finally successful technologies are the crowning end of a 'long and hard journey', after which they become a kind of reward for torments and suffering.

An equally important question is what is excluded from the normalisation limits and what holds a certain potential for social changes.

Lately we can register a certain discursive switch in discussions about reproductive donorship. Both the vocabulary of popular scientific medical and of private and quasi-private ART life stories are framed by free market vocabulary:

> In the Alma-Aty Centre for artificial fertilisation there was a shortage of the main product for this kind of medical institution: sperm. This problem mainly relates to the sperm of Caucasians and Jews, these sperm cells are highly demanded by Kazakhstan's female citizens. (AiF 14.2.2001)

Here market categories such as 'supply and demand' and 'shortage' are used, and donor germ cells are represented as a 'product'. In this discourse, no 'real' life stories are represented. Interestingly, 'sellers' are always men, while 'customers' are, consequently, women. This division of roles is another illustration of the exclusively male genetic retranslation of personal and social characteristics in the media. I consider it as quite important, and of current concern, that these market vocabularies leave a certain freedom and hold potential for transformation and even redefinition of norms related to ARTs. For example, both single women and lesbians, as opposed to a normative nuclear family, are considered potential consumers for the product 'donated sperm'.

Final remarks

In this article, I have tried to analyse how children born with reproductive technologies are problematised, and consequently constituted, in mass-media discourse; how their subjectivities are produced; and how their otherness is made. Russian ART debates are quite heated. The analysed newspaper articles make visible the ambivalent status and contradictory subjectivities of ART children. On the one hand, their otherness is actively produced, which in turn generates early subjectivities of prospective children. With the use of ARTs, an as yet unimplanted embryo becomes personalised, she or he is ascribed identities, rights, and other qualities. Moreover, ART children born with the use of donated biogenetic materials are considered to be a genetic puzzle, and possessing personal and social characteristics that can be designed and constructed according to parents' wishes. The revolutionary potential that these technologies have still generates concerns and fears, in particular, the fear of producing a 'super-human' being with excellent physical, personal and social characteristics. On the other hand – and this is quite logical – ART children are normalised and included into the existing social order. Moreover it is the 'mission' of these children to reconstruct the broken social order, to be included into a modern family concept and to become an 'inheritor', a member in the genetic chain of succession of a family.

The emergence and the wide spread of reproductive technologies by no means constitues a revolution. Notwithstanding public discussion of the possible production of super-human ART children, or transformations of the family – for example, the possibility of reproduction without men – all these novelties are fitted into the regular and established social order in Russian mass media articles. Moreover, these children, and the technologies that made them, are re-oriented and called upon to protect existing forms of kinship and social order. For example, ARTs are interpreted primarily as a way of fighting infertility within a family; but the issue of having a child as a single person or as a lesbian or gay couple is hardly discussed. Another field of the reproduction of the existing social order where the novelty of ARTs is included and normalised are gender relations. They are further represented as constituted by male domination.

In modern public debate on ARTs one can recognise a redefinition of the meaning and status of the human gene. Its meaning exceeds the limits of biomedicine and enables us to talk about the 'geneticisation' of the social. Genes become part of the social worldview. Modern production of subjectivities is connected with genes and with genetic history. ARTs produce a new type of subject whose autonomous status is defined from the moment of conception, whose life story is maintained by genetic history and whose mission it is to ensure genetic continuity.

Notes

[1] Such ideas enable us to decipher the dominant concept of ethnicity in Russian public debates. This is a primordial concept according to which ethnicity is inherited by blood. Moreover, it has a physical expression, it is fixed in the physique. Ethnicity is interpreted as a materialised substance and there are 'carriers' that pass it across generations. A sperm cell acts as such an 'essence carrier'. Thus, ethnicity is localised in a male organism. It is produced and retranslated by a man, which indicates that modern Russian society is a patriarchal one.

References

Brednikova, O. (2008) Dva mira – dva tela? Bestelesnaia sub'ektnost' embriona i bessub'ektnaia telesnost' beremennoi zhenshchiny [Two worlds – two bodies? The 'body-less' subjectivity of the embryo and the 'subject-less' body of the pregnant woman], in N. Nartova and E. Omelchenko (eds) *V Teni Tela* [In the Shadow of the Body]. Ul'yanovsk: Ul'yanovsk State University Press: 113-136.

Conklin, B.A. and Morgan, L.M. (1996) Babies, bodies, and the production of personhood in North America and a Native Amazonian Society, *Ethos,* 24 (4): 657-694.

Dumit, J. and Davis-Floyd, R. (1998) Cyborg babies: children of the third millennium. Introduction, in R. Davis-Floyd and J. Dumit (eds) *Cyborg Babies: From Techno-Sex to Techno-Tots.* New York, London: 1-18.

Franklin, S. (2006) The cyborg embryo: our path to transbiology, *Theory, Culture and Society,* 23(7-8): 167-187.

Haimes, E. (2003) Embodied spaces, social places and Bourdieu: locating and dislocating the child in family relationships, *Body and Society,* 9(1): 11-33.

Haraway, D. (1991) A cyborg manifesto: science, technology, and socialist-feminism in the late twentieth century. In D. Haraway *Simians, Cyborgs and Women: The Reinvention of Nature.* New York: Routledge: 149-181.

Kahn, S. (2004) Eggs and wombs: the origins of Jewishness, in R. Parkin and L. Stone (eds) *Kinship and Family: An Anthropological Reader.* Oxford: Blackwell: 362-377.

Kirejczyk, M. (2008) On women, egg cells and embryos: gender in the regulatory debates on embryonic research in the Netherlands, *European Journal of Women's Studies,* 15(4): 377-391.

Michelle, C. (2007) Human clones talk about their lives: media representations of assisted reproductive and biogenetic technologies, *Media, Culture and Society,* 29(4): 639-663.

Mulkay, M. (1994a) Embryos in the news, *Public Understanding of Science,* 3(1): 33-51.

Mulkay, M. (1994b) Science and family in the great embryo debate, *Sociology,* 28(3): 699-715.

Mulkay, M. (1996) Frankenstein and the debate over embryo research, *Science, Technology and Human Values,* 21(2): 157-176.

Rapp, R. (1991) Moral pioneers: women, men, and fetuses on a frontier of reproductive technology, in M. di Leonardo (ed.) *Gender at the Crossroads of Knowledge: Feminist Anthropology in the Postmodern Era.* Berkeley, Los Angeles, Oxford: University of California Press: 383-395.

Shields, R. (2006) Flanerie for cyborgs, *Theory, Culture and Society,* 23(7-8): 209-220.

Silverman ,D. (1995) *Interpreting Qualitative Data: Methods for Analyzing Talk, Text and Interaction*. London: Sage.

Seguin, E. (2001) Narration and legitimation: the case of in vitro fertilization, *Discourse Society*, 12: 195-215

subRosa (2004) Sex and gender in the biotech century biomediale, in D. Bulatov (ed.) *Contemporary Society and Genomic Culture*. Kaliningrad: The National Publishing House 'Yantarny Skaz', http://biomediale.ncca-kaliningrad.ru/?blang=eng&author=subrosa (last accessed July 4, 2009).

Thacker, E. (2004) Darwin's waiting room, in D. Bulatov (ed.) *Contemporary Society and Genomic Culture*. Kaliningrad: The National Publishing House 'Yantarny Skaz', http://biomediale.ncca-kaliningrad.ru/?blang=eng&author=subrosa (last accessed July 4, 2009).

Zdravomyslova, E. (2009) Gendernoe grazhdanstvo i abortnaia kul'tura [Gendered citizenship and the culture of abortion], in E. Zdravomyslova and Temkina (eds) *Zdorov'e i doverie: Gendernyi podkhod k rerpoduktivnoi medicine* [Health and Trust: A Gender Approach to Reproductive Medicine]. St. Petersburg: European University in St. Petersburg Press: 108-135.

Medical scientific discourse and reproductive genetics

Fertility science-as-culture: ambiguous nature, quantified abstractions and the making of normality

Shahanah Schmid

The sociological and anthropological study of ARTs has generally drawn upon, as its prime materials, ethnographic interviews and observations, as well as documents available in the media and from legislative processes. In this chapter, I present an analysis that uses an approach similar to that of many previous studies, but I have applied it to slightly different materials, enabling new and different kinds of insights. One of the strengths of social science research on technologies of assisted reproduction (ARTs) has been its multi-disciplinarity. Coming from different disciplinary backgrounds, researchers have approached these topics with a multitude of methods, and have studied numerous different kinds of materials. These materials include utterances – be they obtained by ethnographic interviews, participant observation, or the study of published documents – which I roughly categorise into four groups of people. First, there are people not directly involved, but commenting on ARTs;[1] second, people regulating ARTs; third, people undergoing ARTs; and finally, people who research and practice ARTs. Materials derived from all four groups have provided the basis for rich analysis. However, I find it striking that although fertility scientists and practitioners – the fourth group of people – have often been interviewed and observed, there is little social science research based on their publications. There is, of course, the work by Bettina Bock v. Wülfingen (2007, and this volume), who productively uses articles published by fertility experts; however, these are articles in lay magazines, addressing a lay public. Inspired by Emily Martin's (1991) seminal 'Egg and Sperm' paper, I have turned my attention to the scientific publications by Swiss fertility researchers and practitioners. In the following, I will analyse and discuss the discourse in such scientific publications, not asking if they are objectively correct or which facts they convey, but how they create normality, and what kind of normality that is. This constitutes a cultural analysis of these texts.

Obviously such an approach must assume that there is indeed something 'cultural' about scientific publications. Indeed, this is not really debated; on the contrary, there is so much about science that can be seen as culture, that it becomes necessary to define what kind of culture is meant. I follow Marilyn Strathern's (1992b: 33) understanding of culture:

> Culture consists in the way analogies are drawn between things, in the way certain thoughts are used to think others. Culture consists in the images which make imagination possible, in the media with which we mediate experience.

Thus, culture is not about what we think, but rather about how we think. It is important to stress that the culture I am scrutinising here is not the 'science culture' as propagated by Karin Knorr Cetina (2002), that is to say the subtle ways in which procedures, techniques, forms of collaboration and styles of writing interactively create 'facts' and 'knowledge'. In Sarah Franklin's (1995b) terms, Knorr Cetina's science cultures could be described as cultures *of* science. Whilst this is surely of interest, my project, similar to Martin's (1991), lies more in exploring science *as* culture. Science and culture are thus not conceived as separate spheres. The cultural analysis of scientific discourses which follows is part and parcel of general cultural analysis. The focus lies not so much on what the material reveals about scientific ways of knowing and thinking (cultures *of* science), but rather on what scientific discourse tells us about how we all think and know things (science *as* culture).

A note and a caveat on the 'Swissness' of my material and interpretations are needed. 'There is no national science just as there is no national multiplication table; what is national is no longer science,' goes a famous quote by Anton Chekhov. Does it make sense to claim to be analysing Swiss, rather than universal, science-as-culture? At the present stage, I cannot give a definite answer to this question. However, there are reasons to believe that Chekhov might have been wrong. For instance, many academics have pointed out that research is always dependent on the person(s) doing it – their political and ideological backgrounds (Said 1978), their standpoint (Harding 1986), and their social status and origin (Bourdieu 1993) – all of which relates to, and the latter obviously includes, nationality. Thus a science-as-culture which is nationally diversified remains at least a possibility. Further, the aura of universality pertaining to science derives to a large extent from an assumed universality of science's object, nature. Yet, as Anna Lowenhaupt Tsing (1995: 114) points out, 'Nature, like God, is both lawful and mysterious; it requires human efforts to know it, yet always slips away from full knowledge.' This tension between universal nature and nature as wild, varying and unruly is exactly where the cultural specificity of nature as an object of knowledge lies, she argues.

On the other hand, there is a strong argument for increasing global standardisation of science. Whereas scholars used to study foreign languages in order to be able to read fellow academics' papers, nowadays the standard language of publication is English. Scientists travel around the world to pursue their careers, and nationally based journals are threatened with obscurity in the face of publications such as 'Nature' and 'Science'. With the science job market being very international, the more we have scientists working and publishing in countries other than those where they grew up, the harder it should be to detect 'national' inflections in their work. Still, having restricted my material to publications by authors working at Swiss fertility clinics, I will refrain from making generalised statements about science and refer to 'Swiss science'. The reason being, apart from wanting to err on the side of caution, that medicine is yet much less globalised than 'pure' science. Medicine is more regulated by national legislation than other sciences; and since practicing medicine usually requires national licensing, the international mobility of its practitioners is much more restricted.

Methods and materials

The empirical material used consists of six publications, authored by proponents of the three main university hospital fertility clinics in German-speaking Switzerland: one from Zurich; two from Berne; and three from Basle. These are all academic research articles which appeared in peer-reviewed medical journals, four in Swiss journals – three in *Swiss Medical Weekly,* and one in *Journal für Fertilität und Reproduktion* (the Journal for Fertility and Reproduction) – and two in an international journal, *Human Reproduction.* Five of the six papers appeared in English, the sixth provides an English-language abstract. These publications appeared between 2003 and 2007. In this section, I introduce and briefly summarise the content of these six articles. Readers who are uninterested in the technical and scientific sides of ARTs may wish to skip this part.

The article by B. Imthurn from Zurich (Imthurn, Achermann et al. 2004) is a clinical case description of a woman who had experienced repeated miscarriages after IVF conceptions and then came to their clinic. It describes how the doctors applied the procedure of polar body biopsy and thus were able to discard oocytes with aneuploidies. After treatment, the woman successfully bore a healthy child. The article also discusses the legal situation concerning pre-implantation genetic diagnosis (PGD) in Switzerland and abroad, and makes arguments for the legalisation of PGD. There are two articles by C. de Geyter from Basle. The first (de Geyter 2003) is a report of several clinical studies on how ovaries react to hormones during stimulation treatment. It demonstrates that not all ovaries are similarly amenable to these treatments. Since different treatment strategies should be used for different ovaries, the article argues for better diagnostic tools and, consequently, for individualised instead of standardised treatment. De Geyter's second paper (De Geyter, De Geyter et al. 2006) reports a study in which babies' birth weights were measured and compared to the manner of their conception. This paper's novelty lies in the chosen reference group: babies not drawn from the general population, but rather those conceived naturally by women who had 'previously been infertile'. It shows significantly lower birth weights for babies conceived with the help of ART, but only if delivered prematurely; and discusses possible reasons for this finding. The third article from Basle was authored by M. de Geyter, C. de Geyter's wife. This paper (de Geyter, Steinmann et al. 2007) is both a clinical case description as well as a report on a prospective study, involving freezing and thawing of un-inseminated oocytes. It demonstrates that the chosen method of cryo-preserving egg cells has unsatisfactory results, and describes the case of the only successful birth of a baby achieved during the study – nonetheless the first of its kind in Switzerland. Finally from Berne, I have included two articles by D. Wunder and her team, although in one of them she is but the second author. The first (Wunder, Limoni et al. 2005), uses a large set of aggregated statistical data collected by the federal bureau of statistics to examine the question of seasonal influences on IVF procedures on a scale which promises statistically robust results. It is not a clinical study, but a re-examination of statistical data. The findings do not support any seasonal influences, and thus the paper recommends not adapting IVF treatments to specific seasons. The second paper (Crazzolara, Wunder et al. 2007) discusses results from studying sperm quality of fertile men, with the aim of establishing better criteria for when ART treatment is recommended and when it is not. Its conclusions are vague, claiming that no single sperm property is predictive of fertility, but rather a combination of several criteria is 'probably' more useful.

The papers were selected by searching for ARTs practitioners in German-speaking Switzerland, who also conduct research. I used the PubMed database of medical journal publications, browsed the clinicians' homepages, and looked through specifically Swiss journals related to ARTs. Whereas most reproductive physicians did some research at some time, I only found new publications from practitioners who are located at university hospitals. From the results, I selected those papers that were directly relevant to ARTs, and were recently published. These are all scientific texts and use highly specialised language. They are adapted to certain disciplinary standards and traditions, and are addressed not to the general public, nor patients or politicians, but specifically to other researchers or practitioners in the field. They were peer-reviewed before publication and thus necessarily conform to standards of publication in medical journals.

As explained above, I attempted a cultural analysis of this material, with a strong focus on how and what kind of normality is created. I explore the agency of these discourses in creating effects of normality, rather than the intentions of the authors. The authors obviously strongly intended to create a text which adheres to the standards of publication – standards which include the necessity of the non-standard, that is to say of newness, of reporting some sort of insight which was previously unknown. In so doing, they follow and at the same time reconfirm this particular culture-of-science. Although this would also be an interesting project, I tried to avoid analysing how the discourses create the effects of scientificity, objectivity, and publishability. Unintentionally, however, they also create and represent science-as-culture – and thus these scientific texts are open to cultural analysis. To tackle this task, I started by borrowing 'tools' from critical discourse analysis: suspension of belief; critical reading; open coding and free association; followed by extracting objects and subjects of the discourse (e.g. Gill 2000); and finally, focusing on the interpretation of how normality is created. At first I worked with three of the six papers only (de Geyter 2003; Imthurn, Achermann et al. 2004; Wunder, Limoni et al. 2005). This resulted in some interesting hypotheses and insights. I then turned to the other three papers in order to verify if these insights could be found in the new articles and if different issues might come up. In the following, however, I present the results in an integrated manner, and interwoven with interpretation and analysis.

Abstract quantities

When first I familiarised myself with these documents, it was a strange world indeed into which I was immersing myself. It is a world in which abstract concepts sometimes develop more agency than people – questions arise, findings persist, and variables decide, but people are more likely to postpone decisions, if they are visible at all. This invisibility of people largely includes the authors of the text as well – the doers of the experiments, the observers of the cases reported. This world has little to do with the world of medicine we all know from seeing our doctors, where real people get together in real places and do concrete things about the pains we feel. It is rather a decidedly scientific world, in which, to be perceived as a subject worth listening to, you should paradoxically never say 'I'; and in which you can gain the most concrete status by discoursing on the most abstract levels. This, of course, was unsurprising; and I put it down to the kind of documents I was reading. It is also the sort of thing I was explicitly not interested in; as explained above, I leave it to other projects to detect how grammatical passive constructions along with certain standards of 'prospectivity' give a text the quality of being publishable in a medical journal. Yet, in order to achieve ethnographic immersion, I had to learn this language and make this way of thinking my own.

So in order to learn the vocabulary, so to speak, of the culture I was trying to study, I made long lists of words – of the subjects and objects found in this discursive world of science. And while I was busy trying to work out the stories these abstract objects tell, without analysing the abstractions too much – this is not what I am interested in, remember – I nearly missed the real relevance the abstractions have for my project.

Under the scientific imperative of abstraction, even the most concrete things tend to be abstracted in some way or other. A pregnancy, for instance, is of little interest; instead, pregnancy rates receive much attention. Hormones are some of the more concrete objects to be found, in contrast to the predominating objects such as variables, outcomes, and data; but even hormones come in concentrations. Even people with attributes are abstracted. Instead of a woman 37 years of age, we encounter a woman who belongs to the group of 35-40 year olds; I call this abstraction by aggregation. This woman is not in treatment because her husband is infertile, but rather because she is a member of the group of people in treatment because of male infertility factor. Struggling with the complex sentences necessitated by such abstractions, which can only appear as absurd to outsiders, I realised that they do more work than just create an effect of scientificity. They also aggregate individuals into groups, fracture items into densities, and change success, which becomes something not for the individuals, but instead found in a rate. All of these abstractions make the concrete item, process or person countable and measurable. This trick not only enables conformity to the scientific demand for methodological rigour, often perceived to lie in quantity and statistical procedure; but also provides the means for taming the unruly, wilful outlier into a neat, statistical mean.

Charis Thompson (2005: 94) identified the 'epistemic culture based on statistics' as an underlying feature of fertility clinics, guiding – and haunting – everyday practices and decisions. Cumulative probabilities based on statistics are notoriously foggy; they will never provide an answer to the question, 'If I try this, will I get pregnant?' As Thompson (2005: 95) states:

> In practice, this epistemic standard is extremely difficult to live with because it disregards mechanism. If the very same thing works only one in five times, then there is no positive answer to the question of the cause and effect of the infertility. This epistemic difficulty is managed on a daily basis so that it doesn't interfere with practice.

At the same time, referring to statistical probabilities – statistification, as de Jong dubs it (see introduction, this volume) – is a versatile tool for legitimising repeated attempts at ARTs. 'Cycles can always be ruled crucially not the same and so not counted; statistics will always say that this might be the time that the same procedure will work,' observes Thompson (2005: 95). In the more abstract scientific culture which I explored, there are similar effects. For instance, when comparing birth weights of children conceived naturally to ARTs babies, De Geyter (2006: 706) simply excludes those cases which could possibly be 'interfering with the aim of the study'; they are different enough to warrant such exclusion. Their difference would interfere with the statistical procedures intended. Thus, statistical procedures shape normality. Difficulties such as twin pregnancies and cases of neonatal death and major physical malformations are marginalised as being not normal enough – not same enough – to be 'counted'. But far from always being excluding, the versatile functionality of statistics also allows inclusiveness by generalisation. The range of concrete people who have different experiences of ARTs – some get pregnant after one treatment cycle, others submit to multiple attempts, and others again, achieve many pregnancies but never bear a child – is captured by a single inclusive number, the mean success rate. Everybody's unique experience is included, whilst at the same time aggregated, de-individualised, and made invisible, by this one statistical indicator. Statistics can thus domesticate the wild, unruly, not-quite-fitting individual case precisely by including it into a generalised term. Thus, from manifold unique cases, generalised by aggregation and statistical evaluation, arises a new kind of normality: the statistical norm.

The culture, or ways of thinking, observed here is not particular to science. As Strathern (1992a: 27) tells us, the problem which is solved by quantification is the general problem of the relationship between the diverse individual and the general. She further argues that

> (…) the question of how one moves from individual cases to generalisations about systems is, so to speak, an indigenous one. (Strathern 1992a: 26)

Although she is referring to the English, this can probably be generalised across Euro-American cultures. Thus, I would claim that we have here an instance where the ways science makes sense of things is exemplary of how non-scientists think as well; of science-as-culture (Franklin 1995b).

The normal and its 'other'

Since poststructuralism and Foucault, we are more than ever aware that the normal and the deviant stand in a constitutive relationship to each other. We have also learned, from Bourdieu (2001) in particular, that often that which is different is more visible than that which is 'same'; the latter having the qualities of doxa, or being founded on shared, unacknowledged and unconscious beliefs which must necessarily remain implicit. The constitutive relationship which the normal has to its deviants can thus be exploited. By studying the more easily accessible deviant, we can find out all sorts of things about the implicit 'normal'. Leaving a static, somewhat structuralist perception behind, we can go a step further: by exploring the deviant in a discourse, for example, we can describe the ongoing constitution of a fluid, changing normality. Thus we research not simply the normal, but also the process of becoming normal, or making the normal, or normalisation.

In the material I studied, it is striking how often, on the grammatical level at least, the standard remains implicit whilst the deviant is clearly mentioned. This is usually achieved by using comparative degrees[2] but no referents. As an illustration, the texts are full of 'lower sperm counts', 'reduced pregnancy rates', and 'poorer maturation', but rarely do we find a 'than'. Hardly ever are we explicitly told, compared to what something is lower, reduced or poorer. Now I should take care not to over-interpret this finding. After all, this is most likely simply an effect of 'statistics-talk'; a language in which relations between variations are key. Where a change in or a different degree of A is associated with a change in or a different degree of B, it is this association which is declared, rather than the differences within A and B. This explains the lack of referents. Still, textbooks on conducting discourse analysis remind us that we should be concerned with 'what is actually said or written, not some general idea that seems to be intended' (Potter and Wetherell as quoted in Gill 2000: 178). Thus encouraged to further inspect the explicit deviants and implicit referents in my material, a pattern emerges: in all but one of the cases I was able to detect in my material, the explicit comparative is 'worse', implying that the implicit referent, the standard, is 'better'.[3] This raises questions as to what exactly is being normalised in these texts. I will discuss this on the basis of some examples.

> The advanced reproductive biological age of the woman goes hand in hand with a reduced susceptibility of the ovaries to the stimulation treatment necessary for IVF or ICSI. (de Geyter 2003: 7)

In this excerpt, not only is there (bad) reduced susceptibility opposed to an unnamed good standard, but also we find the association of being substandard with advanced age. Thus, the combination youth = high fertility = normal is implied. Thus, advanced age is not simply associated with low chances of procreating, but is also implicitly constituted as abnormal. The next example is similar, but interesting due to the peculiar role that nature and human intervention play:

> Furthermore, lower sperm counts in non-treated ejaculate (observed during the summer months) are compensated in IVF treatment cycles by utilizing a concentrated and constant amount of motile sperm to inseminate the oocytes. (Wunder, Limoni et al. 2005: 3123)

In this case, again, lower is mentioned as deviant from an unspecified standard, thus constructing higher sperm counts, or fertility, as the standard referent. Interestingly, the 'high standard' of fertility is associated with human intervention, and the deviant, lower quality is associated with 'non-treated', or natural, ejaculate. Thus, this excerpt demonstrates that the high, good *standard* need not necessarily be the more *natural*. Rather, the unruly natural variations are compensated for, improved, by medical treatment procedures. These are strongly associated with concentration and constancy, perhaps implying control. Thus, subtly, the association of normal = reproductive medicine = high fertility has been created.

In nearly all cases of comparatives in my material, the implicit referent is associated with fertility and/or successful technology. Importantly, however, it does not always imply nature. This points to issues which medicine has with nature which I will explore later. For now, what does it mean that fertility, as well as success in fertility treatment, is normalised? On the one hand, youthful fertility being assumed as long as there is no counter-indication, is something we are familiar with. Heterosexual couples who do not want to have children do not, in general, go to have their fertility tested; rather, they assume fertility and use contraception. With fertility being normal, infertility is deviant, and can become medicalised. This is obviously quite important for practitioners of reproductive medicine: infertility is a problem which has a medical solution. By also normalising ARTs, and, importantly, not relying exclusively on naturalisations for either of these normalisation strategies, questions of fertility and fertility treatment are removed from the normative jurisdiction of the domain of nature. In the words of Sarah Franklin (1995a: 336), the relation between the natural and the cultural order of facts, has been foundational,[4] but is now changing: 'Assistance introduces a new order of facts that destabilise this foundation: these are the natural facts produced by technology.' Nature, it seems, is not what it used to be.

The nature of Nature

Nature is a common reference point in my scientific texts. Invoking nature in order to confer the status of the unproblematic or self-evident is what Thompson terms naturalisation (2005: 81).[5] This kind of naturalisation can be seen as a specific form of normalisation: something is associated with nature, giving it the aura of self-evidence, making it normal. Indeed, and perhaps unsurprisingly, nature is very present in my material. However, as we have already seen in the previous section, nature is not always associated with the normal. This deserves further exploration.

Nature appears in many forms in my material. For example, by referring to 'central Europe' and 'non-equatorial regions' (Wunder, Limoni et al. 2005) rather than to Switzerland, the idea of geographical regions with similar 'natural' conditions is conjured, rather than speaking about a political entity. In another example, the expression 'Die Gewinnung einer größeren Anzahl Oozyten […]' (de Geyter 2003) could perhaps be translated as 'reclamation of a larger number of oocytes' and raises associations of mining. The image appears of women being mined for oocytes, where the referral to nature in this instance includes an association of women with nature – women as a natural resource. Further, simply referring to men and women as males and females, invokes the animal nature of humans. I have found this throughout all texts, although inconsistently. A further, interesting instance of calling upon nature can be found in the strategic inclusion of animals. Wunder (2005) gives a structured literature review which travels from research on animals to research on humans, and from research on variations in unassisted conception rates to research on ARTs conception rates. What 'work' is nature doing in these examples? What problem is referring to nature in these cases possibly the solution to?[6]

By structuring the literature review in this way, the article creates a subtle continuity from unassisted to assisted conception and from animal to human. Thus, human ART appears as something natural, while preserving the distinctiveness of humans from animals and IVF from unassisted conception. Here, I would argue, nature does the work of rendering interference into human procreation as unproblematic. Where women are figured as natural resources, I believe a similar effect is hidden. In this case, perhaps it is the relationship of physicians to patients as a subject-object relationship which is made unproblematic. In the first example, on the other hand, when the text uses geography to invoke nature, nature bears associations of universality and constancy. Bringing nature into the discussion does the work of providing stability to scientific/statistical results, in this case. Overall, things are being naturalised and thus rendered unproblematic, although we might question to what extent this must always imply normalisation.

The final example however, referring to the animal nature of humans, reveals ambiguities. Animals can be domesticated, and thus humanised; but then they come to represent culture more than nature. The nature that animals are often associated with is wild, undomesticated, and uncontrolled (Lowenhaupt Tsing 1995). Is this the same nature that has a normalising function thanks to its association with universality, constancy, and dependability?

A few instances in my material reveal that associating something with nature does not always have the effect, as described by Thompson (2005), of rendering it unproblematic. Nature can also evoke variability and the need for human intervention and control. A simple example for this can be found in the 'seasons' which are at one point described as a possible cause for varying fertility. Assisted reproductive technologies control such variations by inducing technologically controlled constancy (see also the example where ARTs rather than natural conception are set as standard, in the previous section of this article). Male sperm quality is another area where nature is just not quite good enough. The aim of the paper which discusses sperm quality (Crazzolara, Wunder et al. 2007) is to determine the parameters of sperm in fertile men. Usually, however, men's sperm is used to determine their fertility. In turning this relation upside down, new criteria for defining fertility are needed, and this is exactly what nature fails to provide. A laboriously devised new definition is applied in this text: a man is included as fertile in the study only if his partner is currently pregnant, and if this pregnancy was achieved without medical help within a maximum of fifteen months of not using contraception. The unruly natural variations of sperm quality and fertilisation rates need be contained in order to be able to extract the 'natural' parameters of fertile sperm.

Referring to nature solves a different problem in these examples than that which we encountered previously. Here, nature provides legitimacy not for the status quo, but rather for intervention – the same thing which would previously have been called interference. This double nature of nature has long haunted biomedicine. On the one hand, deviation from the natural is, or causes, disease, and thus needs to be remedied by medicine, with the aim of restoring the natural state. On the other hand, nature is wild, unpredictable, and needs to be controlled. Perhaps within ARTs, nature's double nature is most poignantly felt when women's natural cycles are controlled and standardised in order to restore their natural fertility (Thompson 2005: 96-99). What has become clear is, however, that the double nature of nature prevents any simple equation of naturalisation with normalisation, just as no association of nature with unproblematic universals can be assumed.

Concluding reflections

The scientific papers I have studied for this cultural analysis are all presented in a very similar fashion. Each of them begins with an abstract. The articles proper start with an introduction, followed by a section called 'materials and methods'. Thus far, my own writing exactly replicates that pattern. However, the ethnographic work of writing culture does not go well with the clear structuring into 'results' and 'discussion' that is common in scientific papers. Rather, I have tried to interweave observations and interpretations, and to include theoretical investigations wherever they were prompted by the empirical material. Thus, this conclusion is not meant to provide a summary of the results in slightly different words, but to bring together some lines of thought from the different sections.

One thing that has become clear throughout this chapter is that nature is an ambiguous, somewhat slippery concept. Consequently, naturalisation, as a strategy of rendering something unproblematic by associating it with the domain of nature, turns out to be itself problematic. We must ask, which nature, and also, which naturalising, when we study how people strategically employ nature in order to achieve specific effects. In my material, nature is invoked both to imply justification of the status quo by referring to universality, and to justify intervention by bringing up the wild, variable, unruly nature of nature. Thus, I agree with Lowenhaupt Tsing (1995: 114) when she argues that

> (…) we tend to write of 'naturalizing' social relations as a synonym for 'justifying' them, thus ignoring the cultural specificity of the justification through reference to nature.

It follows that the work done by referring to nature is culturally specific. It is as particular to a certain context as referring to religion, civilization, or progress. In the context in which Lowenhaupt Tsing explored nature,

> (…) the work of nature in U.S. American culture is to create the space for a tension between those forms of agency we best know and those we imagine to be outside our ken. (Lowenhaupt Tsing 1995: 114)

This tension is omnipresent in my material. We find nature as the wild and variable versus nature as the domesticated universal, and nature controls (limits, defines) what is culturally possible, whilst at the same time culture (technology) is needed to control it.

Asking the question about nature invokes a similar query about culture. If we assumed a particular constitutive relation between nature and culture, as is often done when Science and Technology Studies (STS) scholars speak of co-construction, then variable nature would mean variable culture, and the concomitant interest often lies in the boundary work. In contrast, Thompson (2005) explores how people strategically employ a whole careful choreography of references to different 'ontological' domains. However, I believe that my investigations of fertility science-as-culture reveal something different than a dance of invoking different ontologies of nature and culture for normalisation purposes. When nature is used for legitimisation in my material (culture is rarely referred to at all), it has a range of different purposes – sometimes normalising, sometimes just the opposite. Thus I would argue that what I observed is an instance of what Franklin (1995a) described as nature having lost its founding power. It is then not simply the boundary between nature and culture that is shifting, but rather, a whole new relation between these two domains is observed. When it was technologically assisted procreation which was found to be normalised in some cases rather than nature, then nature is not what we expected it to be. As Franklin (1995a: 333-334) writes: 'The necessity for technological assistance thus comes to be seen as a product of nature itself.' Technologically enabled nature becomes the new normality. We might see this as the introduction of a different order of knowledge, one which transcends the 'after nature' dependence of culture which was characteristic of Western thought in much of the 20th century (Strathern 1992a). And yet, in science, as in everyday life, we do not observe this different order of knowledge displacing other ways of constructing meaning. They exist in parallel. What has disappeared is, at most, a perceived singularity of knowledge orders, if ever that was the case.

Notes

[1] This is often done by media, and thus studies of the media are an important approach to ARTs. Also relevant, however, is the approach by Edwards (1999 [1993]) who simply conducted ethnographic interviews about ARTs with northern English villagers.

[2] Such comparisons rely on previous quantification, which was the topic of an earlier section in this article.

[3] In many cases, evaluation as good or bad is not found directly in the comparative, as these tend to be strictly quantitative: more, less, higher, lower, reduced, increased. However, closer inspection revealed that they were always associated with an outcome which was more or less explicitly negative, such as less success, less pregnancies, more disabilities, more deaths.

[4] Foundational is here meant as for figuring kinship, but also, in a wider sense, for culture.

[5] She also mentions the 'rendering of states of affairs and facts in a scientific or biological idiom' as a form of naturalisation. I will disregard this for now, as the biological is very close to natural; and analysing the scientific idiom of scientific papers would imply interpreting what is simply an effect of this kind of text, as having further meanings. This could lead to over-interpretation.

[6] Widdicombe (1993), as summarised by Gill (2000: 180) suggests asking this question as an analytical strategy.

Materials

Crazzolara, S., Wunder, D. et al. (2007) Semen parameters in a fertile Swiss population, *Swiss Medical Weekly*, 2007(137): 166-172.

De Geyter, C., De Geyter, M. et al. (2006) Comparative birth weights of singletons born after assisted reproduction and natural conception in previously infertile women, *Human Reproduction*, 21(3): 705-712.

de Geyter, C. (2003) Therapeutische Strategien bei relativer hypergonadotroper Ovarialinsuffizienz, *Journal für Fertilität und Reproduktion*, 2: 7-14.

de Geyter, M., Steinmann, S. et al. (2007) First delivery of healthy offspring after freezing and thawing of oocytes in Switzerland, *Swiss Medical Weekly*, 137(31-32): 443-447.

Imthurn, B., Achermann, J. et al. (2004) Preimplantation diagnosis in Switzerland: birth of a healthy child after polar body biopsy, *Swiss Medical Weekly*, 134: 259-261.

Wunder, D.M., Limoni, C. et al. (2005) Lack of seasonal variations in fertilization, pregnancy and implantation rates in women undergoing IVF, *Human Reproduction*, 20(11): 3122-3129.

References

Bock v. Wülfingen, B. (2007) *Genetisierung der Zeugung. Eine Diskurs- und Metaphernanalyse reproduktionsgenetischer Zukünfte.* Bielefeld: transcript Verlag.

Bourdieu, P. (1993) Narzisstische Reflexivität und wissenschaftliche Reflexivität, in E. Berg und M. Fuchs (Hg.) *Kultur, soziale Praxis, Text: Die Krise der ethnographischen Repräsentation.* Frankfurt am Main: Suhrkamp: 365-374.

Bourdieu, P. (2001) *Meditationen: Zur Kritik der scholastischen Vernunft.* Frankfurt am Main: Suhrkamp.

Edwards, J. ([1993] 1999) Explicit connections: ethnographic enquiry in northwest England, in J. Edwards, S. Franklin, E. Hirsch, F. Price and M. Strathern (eds) *Technologies of Procreation: Kinship in the Age of Assisted Conception.* London: Routledge: 60-85.

Franklin, S. (1995a) Postmodern procreation: a cultural account of assisted reproduction, in F. Ginsburg, and R. Rapp (eds) *Conceiving the New World Order: The Global Politics of Reproduction.* Berkeley: University of California Press: 323-345.

Franklin, S. (1995b) Science as culture, cultures of science, *Annual Review of Anthropology*, 24: 163-184.

Gill, R. (2000) Discourse analysis, in M.W. Bauer and G. Gaskell (eds) *Qualitative Researching with Text, Image and Sound.* London: Sage: 172-190.

Harding, S. (1986) *The Science Question in Feminism.* Ithaca: Cornell University Press.

Knorr Cetina, K. (2002) *Wissenskulturen. Ein Vergleich naturwissenschaftlicher Wissensformen.* Frankfurt am Main: Suhrkamp.

Lowenhaupt Tsing, A. (1995) Empowering nature, or: some gleanings in bee culture, in S. Yanagisako and C. Delaney (eds) *Naturalizing Power: Essays in Feminist Cultural Analysis.* New York, London: Routledge: 113-143.

Martin, E. (1991) The egg and the sperm, *Signs,* 16(3): 485-501.

Said, E.W. (1978) *Orientalism.* London: Routledge and Kegan Paul.

Strathern, M. (1992a) *After Nature: English kinship in the late twentieth century.* Cambridge: Cambridge University Press.

Strathern, M. (1992b) *Reproducing the Future: Essays on Anthropology, Kinship and the New Reproductive Technologies.* Manchester: Manchester University Press.

Thompson, C. (2005) *Making Parents: The Ontological Choreography of Reproductive Technologies.* Cambridge MA, London: MIT Press.

Bridgeheads and concerns in the normalisation of reproductive genetics in Germany

Bettina Bock v. Wülfingen

At the beginning of the third millennium, pressure was high in German politics to develop a new legal framework to fundamentally change the legal uses and regulation of human biotechnology. Many scientific groups were involved, including ambitious German scientists engaged with the Human Genome Project; reproductive physicians who wanted legalisation of preimplantation genetic diagnosis; and stem cell researchers who hoped to work with embryonic material. However, the result of these debates was surprising: the Embryo Protection Act, originally enacted in 1990, was reconfirmed. Though long discussion within German parliament – the Bundestag – produced increased awareness of cloning, only the importing of stem cells was legalised. Regulation remained restrictive. The political process prior to these decisions had been accompanied by heavy media coverage in which experts were invited to explain their visions of future uses for new genetic and reproductive technologies. This article discusses experts' modes of normalising these technologies and whether these experts, who were mostly non-German, found ways to reasonably deal with German concerns in terms of a democratisation of technology.

The material that will be analysed includes experts' articles in German print media during the period of these public debates – 1995 to 2003 – a time when domestic biopolitical change seemed possible, at least to some German journalists. Selection of this period of time follows Graumann's (2002) observation that the ethics debate on human biotechnology in reproduction, especially on cloning, started in Germany around 1997 with the birth of Dolly the sheep. To examine normalisation procedures in these texts, I use the bridgehead concept, as introduced by Weingart (1989) in *Technologie als sozialer Prozess,* Technology as a Social Process. Bridgeheads are categories which are stressed in discourses accompanying the introduction of technologies that also strategically connect new technologies with categories and issues which are already part of familiar repertoires within local discourses.

Material for this analysis is drawn from the largest-selling national magazines and high-quality newspapers, which are also read by politicians and media personnel themselves: *Frankfurter Rundschau*; *Frankfurter Allgemeine Zeitung*; *Stern; Die Zeit; Süddeutsche Zeitung; Focus;* and *Der Spiegel* (Informationsgemeinschaft zur Verbreitung von Werbeträgern 2000). Articles from best-selling popular science magazines *Geo* and *Spektrum der Wissenschaften*, from the feminist journal *EMMA,* and the philosophy journal *Ethica*, are also included. A previous study involved macroanalysis of approximately 1,000 publications which matched keywords such as cloning, laboratory reproduction, in vitro fertilisation and preimplantation genetic diagnosis (Bock v. Wülfingen 2007). This overview study mainly contained reports on stem cell policies and cloning debates from a critical perspective. From that large original sample, 30 articles were selected for more in-depth analysis to present an argument in favour of relaxating German regulation of these technologies.

This article is concerned with how ideas about more general uses of combined genetic and reproductive technologies were explained and normalised in German public debates. My analysis aims to discover which locally contingent discursive objects were tackled by experts, and how they dealt with the German context and local concerns. To achieve that aim, it was necessary to examine what kinds of bridgeheads were employed, and what concerns were addressed in these texts; furthermore, the question of whether these bridgeheads were successful in communicating with the public was also important. Finally, this chapter will conclude with a discussion of how, or if, gaps between experts' conceptualisations of the future of reproduction – via cloning, for example – and individuals' emotionally laden notions of reproduction can be bridged.

Normalisation and bridgeheads

The importance of the local contexts in the construction of scientific and medical knowledge is one of the corner stones of Science and Technology Studies. Technologies change from market to market depending on local conditions. They are adapted in different ways by local populations (Fujimura 1997; Latour and Woolgar 1986; Rabinow 1999). National differences in policy processes also have important consequences for definitions related to genetic technologies (Parthasarathy 2004). Concerning new genetic technologies, it has been revealed that a variety of locally and historically contingent discourses of concern prevail in different countries, and that such discourses shape local legal frameworks (Lassen and Jamison 2006). To ensure the success of supply-driven and highly regulated genetic and medical technologies, these discourses of concern must be addressed when these services are introduced into new markets (Etzinga 1998; Lassen and Jamison 2006). Bridgeheads are categories which ease the introduction of new technologies by connecting them to traditions and familiar discourses.

The importance of these discourses of concern and local legal frameworks is especially important with respect to Germany because German legislation bans any treatment of a fertilised egg cell or storage of an embryo. Therefore, it is necessary to investigate genetic reproductive technology and stem cell research as integrated issues in this context. Moreover, the material selected for this study reflects common ground between stem cell research and reproductive genetics in the discussion of their common research infrastructure; shared scientific topics; and similar obstacles to research, such as legal restrictions on access to human genome data and reproductive material. This article assesses experts' discourses in light of these frictions between restriction and expansion; specifically, the expansion of markets, access to human biological material and the crucial extension of experts' competence as a tool to broaden access to biological material and markets. I also draw on the role of local histories and language differences as factors which limit the expansion of technology. This is explained by Anderson (1991), who uses the example of the book and its standardising and universalising effects which promoted the extension of markets. He claims that language differences and orally transmitted local memories – of local heroes, resistance or victims – had to be reduced before larger nations could be built.

Within the German cultural context, it was experts[1] who were given the role of normalising new (or combined) genetic and reproductive technologies by the media. In the health systems of risk societies, these experts perform the task of translating risk knowledge into reproductive choices for families and society (Ettorre 1999; Samerski 2002). While dealing with clients, experts accomplish the quest for normality and rituals (Kolip 2000). The separation of the social from the natural science is one of the major aspects of this difference between expert and layperson. This separation serves the existential maintenance of professional hegemony over the claimed field of expertise. At the same time, experts' interaction with the public sphere is crucial for securing the continuity of genetic science. Securing experts' competence therefore requires a shift from a practical to a theoretical and speculative take on science (Jonsen 1996: 11). The increasing frequency of bioethic committees' calls for experts' translations of science into socially comprehensible language fosters natural scientists' positions in such committees or as writers and commentators in newspapers and journals.

Thus, this article explores the issues and modes of translation which surface in public statements by experts with regard to an apparently promising future of reproductive genetics in Germany. The political context in which these articles appeared constitutes a pivotal moment at the end 1990s, a time of increasing openness and desire for more liberal legislation on human biotechnologies. The next section presents the main findings in this analysis of expert discourses, with a particular focus on how particular local concerns were addressed in the introduction of new genetic and reproductive technology in German print media. The second section view these results with respect to strategies of normalisation, describing major problems in matching science and public discourses in the material.

'Universal' bridgeheads and specific German concerns

The analysis of experts' texts promoting new reproductive and genetic technology from the end of the 1990s onward reveals a new connection of two formerly separate reproductive discourses, namely fertilisation technology aimed at 'healing' infertility, and contraceptive technology which is aimed at the prevention of pregnancy. Both merge in the normalisation of infertility and the presentation of laboratory reproduction as a standard reproductive technique. Major proponents for these views outline a future in which young men and women can ask for sterilisation directly after puberty and store their egg cells and sperm for reproduction later, after their major career steps (Silver in Petermann and Paul 1998; Baker 1999; Djerassi in Blech and Traufetter 2002). This discursive connection of antinatalist and pronatalist technologies with genetics, and in some texts, even with cloning, is of central importance for understanding shifts in the framing of health and illness which are also taking place in these publications. Abject bodies (Butler 1993) are depathologised as potential parents via this geneticisation of conception, and integrated into discourses about wishing to have a child. At the same time, the level of genetic control over an envisioned, and thereby embodied, child shifts to the embryo. Thus, older women at the end of the reproductive phase are invited to take their career seriously first and encouraged to have a child later. Singles and gay couples, especially lesbians, are made welcome to use these technologies to reproduce. Additionally, the concept of health-promising features of the child (the genetic equipment of the embryo) shifts over this time period from 1995 to 2003. There is a move from healing concepts towards genetic health resources and the free choice of genes.

Bridgeheads: love and suffering versus risks

Current analysis of discourses related to new genetic reproductive technologies indicates that themes of risk (Beck 1992), responsibility and choice are prominent. This study, contrarily, suggests that in experts' future fictions, human procreation as standardised laboratory conception revolves around categories which have received little attention so far: love, empowerment and suffering (Bock v. Wülfingen 2007). Empowerment refers to life chances and the genetic optimisation of a child in a competitive society. Love refers to the intimate love between partners as well as to love towards a (future or potential) child. In short, these new discursive structures introduce the 'subject genetically at risk' (Novas and Rose 2000) to the German public with a positive identity instead of fear-inducing connotations. Love and empowerment might work well to normalise reproductive genetic technologies in postindustrial cultures where individual autonomy is a relevant category and where romantic love fulfills the need for intimacy (Luhmann 1986). When compared with love and empowerment, the prevention of suffering seems, initially, to be the most conservative and promising 'universal' bridgehead for introducing reproductive genetic technologies in Germany. The suffering so prevented is that of a future human being afflicted with genetically induced health impairments, and the anguish of involuntarily childless couples. In Germany, however, acceptance of suffering has a long tradition in religion, especially Lutheran and Calvinist traditions following Augustinus, which have been revived by Schleiermacher (Weber [1920] 2000; Hick 1970). Acceptance of suffering, and its positive, educational potential to 'deepen' character is also a theme in philosophy; medicine; critical thinking; the feminist health movement (Beck-Gernsheim 2000; Illich 1975); and in Nietzsche's (1982: 14) critique of medicine. Thus it seems that within German discussions of biomedicine, the acceptance of suffering is comparatively high and, in this context, might not serve well as a bridgehead to normalise morally contested technology (Bock v. Wülfingen 2009). However, there are other normalising procedures that address locally specific concerns rather than attempting to find universal bridgeheads.

According to analysed material, the status of embryos and eugenics are major concerns in Germany. Aware that these matters are a major concern in the German discursive context, some foreign experts *explicitly* tackled them in their optimistic future visions of new reproductive genetic technologies. Such experts presented different features of eugenics, trying to distance their scientific work from any such aims or results. Following one discursive stream, the term eugenics only applies if the germ line, and therefore future generations, were to be affected by genetic manipulations (Hughes 2000; Stock 2000: 192).

> The ghost of eugenics appears again (…). If we manipulate embryos in order to prevent illnesses, won't we go further and strive for the 'optimisation' of human abilities? (Green 1999: 65)

Another position did not differentiate between germ line or soma gene therapy. The definition of eugenics in this case was that the genetic change served the aim of 'enhancing' genes instead of just curing or saving people from illness (Wilmut 2002, 2001; Hughes 2000, Reich 1999).

> Finally one could want to change the genetic equipment of future generations, independent of whether it had to do with illnesses, which is where we enter eugenics. (Reich 1999)

A third position maintained that genetic manipulations were not eugenic acts as long as they did not imply limitations of reproductive liberty:

> This is not about restrictions of reproductive liberty, which would be classical eugenics, but about broadening reproductive options. (Silver in Petermann and Paul 1998: 145)

The embryo of public concern

In the material analysed there is a crucial distinction between technically produced embryos – which are meant to be implanted and gestated, although they are technically clones in some of the expert fictions – and those which are not produced for reproductive means. A new term, activated egg cell, was created in 2001 by the private company Advanced Cell Technology (ACT), and subsequently appeared in the German media. In ACT laboratories, two techniques were used to produce clones. The first method was the electrical stimulation of an egg cell, which produces an activated egg cell. The second method employs the technique used in the production of Dolly: somatic cell nuclear transfer. This technique was used to produce cellular formations which were described as the 'first successful human clone', though these results remain in dispute amongst scientists (Cibelli et al. 2002). Later, in an article published in Germany, an ACT bioethicist presented the following argument:

> Although the [ethics] council was able to understand why some people would equate this tiny organism with an embryo, we preferred the concept of an 'activated egg cell'. Its properties (…) do not justify a prohibition of its use in research which, in the end, could save the lives of children and adults. (Green 2002: 17)

These properties were also discussed by other experts with regard to their origin as well as to their developmental potential: 'You don't create a new genome like when sperm and egg cell amalgamate' (Solter 2002: 23; see also Green 2002: 17). It thus results in a 'completely new type of entity which never existed before in nature' (Green 2002: 17). Additionally 'this product could not develop into a creature' (Solter 2002: 23) and if it could, 'this was only true in a very limited way' (Green 2002: 17). One expert concluded, with respect to German legislation:

> If the blastocyte does not result from the merging of a sperm and an egg cell and since the product can't develop into a living organism (…) it should thus, according to the current German legal framework, be possible to produce such blastocytes for research. (Solter in Epping 2002: 23)

In contrast to this distinction between that which is 'naturally conceived' and an apparent 'technical product', similar differentiations were not made when reproductive cloning was at issue. Such ideas were brought into German media via interviews with, and essays by, non-German scientific experts. Reproductive cloning, which represents the limites of what is acceptable, is not only defended by those who take up this role, which I choose to call that of an anti-hero; but also by others who are marked in the texts as reputable scientists on the basis their careers in state universities. In references to cloned cells meant for reproduction, the parallel between technical cloning and natural processes was highlighted. An article in *Der Spiegel* provided a most salient example in which – this time – the ACT ethicist is not presented as a member and interested ethicist of the private gene-mapping company, but rather as a researcher who literally described the gestated human clone as sibling. This analysis reveals that by 2002, experts more frequently admitted that boundaries between therapeutic and reproductive cloning were blurry, most obviously with respect to gene therapy applied to pregestational embryos (Wilmut 2002: 43).

Using bridgeheads and addressing concerns: do they match local discourses?

Often when new technologies are introduced, discursive bridgeheads are used to link these innovations to existing discourses in order to extend their appeal in a given market. In the introduction of new genetic reproductive technologies in Germany, two vareties of bridgehead were employed: those that address major categories of 'universal' human interest and those that relate to locally-specific concerns. While Lassen and Jamison (2006) find that, with reference to genetic technologies, barriers to acceptance by lay audiences are often believed to be ignorance and lack of information, our findings strongly suggest that most of the experts in our study material also deal with local issues. However, it is still unclear whether experts are able to adequately convince and reassure lay audiences, and whether local concerns are adequately matched with categories chosen as bridgeheads.

The embryo

Terminologies are a crucial part of experts' knowledge cultures. Differences in knowledge of and competence with these vocabularies creates in- and out-groups and specific identities – 'scientific' and 'lay' or 'public' – via discursive delimitations, while also creating the realms of experts' influence. Flexible boundaries set up by terminologies are productive for the creation of particular sciences within science. As Hauskeller (2005: 45) states, the current disputes about 'more or less morally neutral words fix out-dated ideological barriers between biomedical research as a proper 'objective' science and society as its value-laden counterpart.' An important finding by Hauskeller (2005) for bridgeheads and concern-related discursive strategies discussed in this text, is that there are major differences between the United Kingdom and Germany in the usage and problematisation of terms. In the United Kingdom, 'embryoid' or 'embryonic body' never had any similar semantic impact in public discourses or the press (Hauskeller 2005). This phenomenon could be interpreted as a consequence of different regulatory regimes adopted by Germany and Britain to address ethical problems and concerns around embryo research (Hauskeller 2004), which are, in turn, connected to different historical backgrounds of each country. The concept of the embryo is crucial within the German legal framework through the Embryo Protection Act. The British Human Fertilisation and Embryology Act (HFE) – set up in 1990 like the German Embryo Protection Act – allows research on embryos until the fourteenth day of development; however, German legislation protects the embryo from the time of conception. This difference in dealing with the embryo is also reflected in the analysed texts.[2]

Hauskeller (2005) gives an overview of different categories and titles for embryos and embryo-like structures which are disputed between science and the public, such as 'pre-embryo' – a term introduced as early as the 1980s – 'blastocyste' and 'embryoid body'. She stresses that use of these terms in laboratories often far preceded public debates on embryo-ethics. Her finding is that a differentiation between 'reproductive' and 'therapeutic cloning' as well as the notion of 'somatic cell nuclear transfer' (see below) was 'indeed merely strategic' in order to address public concerns (Hauskeller 2005). Other terms, such as blastocyste, refer to an entity which, in daily laboratory work, serves to sharply differentiate the cell body from other conceptualisations of embryonic phases. The concept of the embryoid body was not intended to be used for public representation, and German researchers especially regretted its escape into the public because the term lead to confusion (Hauskeller 2005). Although, in the analytic material, promoters of genetics in reproductive technology recognised this crucial issue within the context of the Embryo Protection Act, their arguments are not congruent with mainstream German perspectives. In a major part of the analysed texts, the ability of the embryo to develop (into a creature) was set as a measure to differentiate technologically processed products from embryos protected by any law. This means that a chain of signification is projected, leading from the embryo via its 'potential to develop' directly into a human being. As explained above, this implied (biological) logic does not stand on firm ground, and is better explained as having been induced by legal conditions that invite us to avoid the notion of the embryo. A potential cloned blastocyte would thereby be exonerated from humanness and the connected ethical issues (Düwell and Mieth 2000). Comments by some experts, even among the articles which promote a more liberal approach to new genetic and reproductive technologies, suggest that separating reproductive clones and clones for therapeutic purposes is difficult to maintain with biological arguments (Wilmut 2002). In 2003, three major political parties in the German parliament decided not to follow this distinction and urged the government not to do so either:

> The forms of cloning of humans and human embryos known to this day, reproductive cloning and so-called therapeutical cloning, are identical until the decision is taken whether they shall be implanted or used for the extraction of stem cells. Thus this does not allow for a distinction between reproductive cloning and so-called therapeutical cloning. The difference only lies in the purpose of the cloning. (Deutscher Bundestag 2003)

Similar arguments were presented during debates on new stem cell research legislation in 2002. Embryos were finally defined as such under the Embryo Protection Act to include *all* entities from the day of conception onward (Deutscher Bundestag 2002).

Since only a small part of the German parliament represents the interests of religious Germans, it is doubtful whether the Embryo Protection Act and later decisions refer to any moral status of the embryo in a religious sense, but rather religious common sense is used for setting a voluntary boundary. Considering the trends of discourse from 1995-2003, it can be seen that German politicians, as well as most expert journalists, are aware that these choices are not rational, but are following Christian ethics by explicitly setting the starting point of human life at conception. The embryo is not defined by future functions or abilities, or the present (non-)differentiation of organs, but by a categorical decision. Since this does not follow any utilitarian logic, those arguments which try to rationally weigh the suffering of adults versus the structure of several cells do not work well. Such arguments are also unsuccessful because of the particular context of German history, that is to say the memory of pervasive rational organisation and relativism with regard to the worth of any human life during the National Socialist period.

> It is like this: the experience we had with German National Socialism, especially with respect to research and science, has to play a major role in ethical decision making (…). We don't remember it because we want to be more moral than all the others. No. The point is not a special German morality. (…) The memory of it is a continuous reminder: nothing must be above the dignity of the individual human being. (then president, Johannes Rau, SPD 2001)

The overwhelming amount of sophisticated scientific studies that discuss *biological* and *ethical* definitions and the status of an embryo seem to indicate that these issues receive major attention in Germany; however the decision of the Bundestag not to take on a flexible utilitarian position can be understood as the utmost delimitation of a *historical* period.

Eugenics

The articles investigated in microanalysis revealed that experts detected the memory of eugenics as a major hindrance for the acceptance of genetics in new reproductive technologies within German culture. As shown above, a variety of concepts of eugenics already exist among experts on new reproductive technologies and this variety becomes even greater when taken together with those understandings of eugenics which are prevalent in German politics or in the public. Graumann (1999) defines such understandings as biological, historical and socio-cultural notions of eugenics, framings which can and should be separated. She traces the root of the biological notion of eugenics back to Francis Galton (1883). In introducing the notion of eugenics, he referred to a material change, or improvement, of heritable factors in a population. Thus the dispersion of features which supposedly had a negative effect on the whole population could be restricted (negative eugenics) and the dispersion of effects deemed to be positive for the population could be enhanced (positive eugenics). Central to this concept is the material changeability of whole populations by selecting properties deemed worthy of reproduction. Additionally, this notion is normative since it refers to a ranking of the quality of properties.

Within the analysed material, three different (biological) notions of eugenics were presented in explanations of potential enhancements in the life chances and conditions of one's offspring. In the first of these conceptualisations, eugenics was only considered as such when reproduction was restricted. This was in contrast to the aim of new reproductive and genetic technologies. This definition, eugenics as reproductive restrictions for some, equals Galton's notion of negative eugenics. The second position amongst experts suggested that all cases of germ line gene therapy which do not aim to prevent illness could be called eugenics. This idea of enhancing genes can be subsumed in Galton's positive eugenics. According to a third permutation, eugenics is always a given when more than one individual is affected by genetic change, which is the case in germ line therapy. This is the description most akin to Galton's concept of eugenics as a whole, since it refers to differences between changing the individual versus changing parts of the population. The latter only happens implicitly in the other descriptions. None of these interpretations refer to the normative character of Galton's concept, according to which it is possible to have consensus about desirable characteristics. However, all these interpretations, including the one by Galton himself, assume that a secured result of the reproductive or genetic manipulation is achievable, thus resulting in the idea of a preplanned somatic expression of this manipulation.

In contrast to these conceptualisations, gene-critical discourse – which was explicitly discussed in German media alongside the ethical debates on human reproductive genetics (Graumann 1999) – relies on a historical or socio-cultural perspective on eugenics which differs significantly from the framings described above. From this perspective, eugenics is the name of a socio-cultural project in which biological sciences having a decisive role and within which science, ideology and demography form a synergistic complex (Meier-Seethaler 1997). According to this point of view, eugenics is a socio-cultural phenomenon of regulation through science, politics and the 'mass consciousness' (Beck-Gernsheim 2000), or it becomes a result of self-discipline and heteronomy framed in the concept of governmentality (Graumann 1999). These authors refer to the historical experience of violence, especially during the National Socialist regime and its continuities. Thus, a profound mismatching results between Anglo-Saxon biological ideas of eugenics, which follow Galton, when they meet discourses of concern relating to the violence of a historical experience of eugenic practices in Germany.

Conclusions

Different local contexts, differences in culture and in history shape national legislation on science and technology research, development and application as well as the overall acceptance of specific technologies. These local differences seem to be in conflict with the expansion of technology if the latter simply relies on 'universal' language and meanings. As Anderson (1991) writes, it is 'specific amnesias', particularly the forgetting of local differences, which enables the expansion of a market which stabilises itself on common characteristics within the thus expanded community. Historically contingent national differences are in part shaped by specific local concerns with regard to specific technologies to which experts refer. With a growing awareness of the need for public understanding of science, experts are challenged to extend their field of competence beyond the limits of their professions. The discursive techniques applied in the analysed material embrace references to categories believed to be universal, of which suffering is the most prominent. Also, locally disputed issues, such as the status of the embryo and eugenics, were detected as problematic categories and explicitly tackled. The use of the category of suffering falsely takes for granted that it has negative connotations, or that it is something every human would want to avoid. Its use as a bridging category in introducing reproductive genetic technology in Germany is therefore likely to fail. This example shows the urgent need to question the universality of some categories and 'humanist' values.

The concept of the embryo is a hotly debated topic in most Christian countries, even more so in Germany because of the Embryo Protection Act which forbids any usage of fertilised egg cells apart from implantation. This complicates differentiation between 'therapeutic' and 'reproductive' cloning. Additionally, the notion of eugenics, which is not found to be an issue to the same extent in any other country, has been detected by experts as a concern which, in the German context, had to be addressed when talking of human genetics. Some experts' texts dealt with the ambivalence of invoking these issues of concern, which brings forth the memory of issues which normalising discourses aim to overcome. Thus these concerns are often immediately trivialised, in the sense of 'let's forget the horror scenarios' (Green 1999: 63). Consequently, this might give the impression that locally-specific memories may simply be forgotten or silenced in order for individuals to get access to seemingly necessary technologies or to extend markets. Thus, experts' discussion of these ideas does not exactly meet core problems within these discussed concerns. However, the analysis of normalisation procedures of (combined) genetic reproductive technologies in Germany shows that universal categories are not the only ones being used discursively. Locally contingent bridgeheads and concerns are spotted and actively addressed too.

Notes

[1] In the terms of Kuhn 1973.

[2] Only one expert within the researched material refers to eugenics (calling it a 'ghost') without distancing himself (Stock 2000: 192).

References

Anderson, B. (1991) *Imagined Communities: Reflections on the Origin and Spread of Nationalism.* London and New York: Verso.

Bahnsen, Ulrich (2000) Wunderbare Kräfte. Mark Hughes hat ein Retortenbaby erzeugt – es soll einem kranken Bruder Knochenmark spenden, *Die Zeit,* 39/2000.

Baker, R. (1999) Der Mensch wird seine Reproduktion bald voll steuern, *Focus,* 22/1999: 163.

Beck-Gernsheim, E. (2000) Health and responsibility: from social change to technological change and vice versa, in B. Adam, U. Beck and J. Van Loon (eds) *The Risk Society and Beyond: Critical Issues for Social Theory.* London: Sage: 122-135.

Beck, U. (1992) *Risk Society: Towards a New Modernity.* London: Sage.

Blech, Jörg und Gerald Traufetter (2002) Laborbabys werden mehr geliebt, *Spiegel,* 4: 76-77.

Bock v. Wülfingen, B. (2007) *Genetisierung der Zeugung.* Bielefeld: transcript-Verlag.

Bock v. Wülfingen (forthcoming 2009) Human genetic technologies in international contexts: a comparison, in *Ethik transdisziplinär: 'Genetic Screening'.* Salzburg.

Butler, J. (1993) *Bodies that Matter: On the Discursive Limits of 'Sex'.* New York: Routledge.

Cibelli, J. B., R. P. Lanza and D. W. Michael (2002) Die ersten geklonten menschlichen Embryonen, *Spektrum der Wissenschaft,* 1: 12-17.

Deutscher Bundestag (2002) Plenarprotokoll 14/211 – Stenographischer Bericht, Deutscher Bundestag, 14. Wahlperiode – 214. Sitzung, 30.01.2002. Berlin: Deutscher Bundestag.

Deutscher Bundestag (2003) Drucksache 15, 15. Wahlperiode, 18.02.2003. Berlin: Deutscher Bundestag.

Djerassi, C. (1999) *Der entmachtete Mann,* EMMA, 5: 50-51.

Düwell, M. and Mieth, D. (2000) *Ethik in der Humangenetik.* Frankfurt am Main: Suhrkamp.

Epping, Bernhard (2002) Lieber gleich die ganze Wahrheit sagen, *Spektrum der Wissenschaft*, 1: 22-23.

Ettorre, El. (1999) Experts as 'storytellers' in reproductive genetics: exploring key issues', *Sociology of Health and Illness,* 21 (5): 539-559.

Etzinga, A. (1998) Theoretical perspectives: culture as a resource for technological change', in A. Hård and A. Jamison *The intellectual Appropriation of Technology: Discourses on Modernity 1900-1990.* Cambridge MA: MIT Press: 21-44.

Franklin, S. (2005), 'Discussion comment' at the Workshop Between the Farm and the Clinic: Agriculture and Reproductive Technology in the Twentieth Century. Cambridge: 29.04.2005.

Fujimura, J. (1997) *Crafting Science: A Sociohistory of the Quest for the Genetics of Cancer.* Cambridge, MA: Harvard University Press.

Galton, F. (1883) *Inquiries into Human Faculty and its Development.* London: Macmillan.

Graumann, S. (2002) Die Rolle der Medien in der Debatte um die Biomedizin, in S. Schicktanz, C. Tannert and P. M. Wiedemann (eds) *Kulturelle Aspekte der Biomedizin: Bioethik, Religionen und Alltagsperspektive.* Frankfurt am Main: Campus: 212-243.

Green, R. M. (1999) Mein Kind ist mein Zwilling, *Spektrum Spezial,* 4: 62-65.

Green, R. M. (2002) Die Ethik des Klonens, *Spektrum der Wissenschaft,* 1: 17-24.

Hauskeller, C. (2004) How traditions of ethical reasoning and institutional processes shape stem cell research in the UK, *Journal of Medicine and Philosophy,* 29/5: 509-532.

Hauskeller, C. (2005) The Language of Stem Cell Science, in W. Bender, C. Hauskeller and Alexandra Manzei (eds.) *Crossing Borders – Grenzüberschreitungen: Ethische, Politische und Religiöse Kontexte der Stammzellforschung.* Münster: Agenda Verlag: 39-60.

Hick, J. (1970) Freedom and the Irenean Theodicy Again, *Journal of Theological Studies,* 21: 419-422.

Illich, I. (1975) *Medical Nemesis: The Expropriation of Health.* London: Marian Boyars.

Informationsgemeinschaft zur Verbreitung von Werbeträgern (2000) IVW Praxis. Bonn: IVW.

Jonsen, A. R. (1996) The impact of mapping the human genome on the patient-physician relationship, in T.H. Murray, M.A. Rothstein and RF. Murray (eds) *The Human Genome Project and the Future of Health Care.* Bloomington: Indiana University Press: 7-11.

Kolip, P. (ed) (2000) *Weiblichkeit ist keine Krankheit: Die Medikalisierung körperlicher Umbruchphasen im Leben von Frauen.* Weinheim, München: Juventa.

Kuhn, T. S. (1973) *Die Struktur wissenschaftlicher Revolutionen.* Frankfurt am Main: Suhrkamp Verlag.

Lassen, J. and Jamison, A. (2006) Genetic technologies meet the public: the discourses of concern, *Science, Technology, & Human Values,* 31(1), 8-28.

Latour, B. and Woolgar, S. (1986) *Laboratory Life: The Construction of Scientific Facts.* Princeton NJ: Princeton University Press.

Luhmann, N. (1986) *Love as passion: The codification of intimacy.* Cambridge: Polity Press.

Meier-Seethaler, C. (1997) *Gefühl und Urteilskraft – ein Plädoyer für die emotionale Vernunft.* München: Beck.

Nietzsche, F. (1982) *Die fröhliche Wissenschaft.* Frankfurt am Main: Insel.

Novas, C. and Rose, N. (2000) Genetic risk and the birth of the somatic individual, *Economy and Society,* 29(4): 485-513.

Petermann, Jürgen und Rainer Paul (1998) Gefährlicher als die Bombe, *Spiegel* (29), 142-145.

Rabinow, P. (1999) *French DNA: Trouble in Purgatory.* Chicago: University of Chicago Press.

Rau, J. (2001) 'Wird alles gut? Für einen Fortschritt nach menschlichem Maß http: //www.bundespräsident.de (accessed Nov. 27, 2008).

Reich, J. (1999) Gentherapie gegen individuelles Leid, *Süddeutsche Zeitung,* 212, V(2): 7 (14.7.1999).

Samerski, S. (2002) *Die verrechnete Hoffnung: Von der selbstbestimmten Entscheidung durch genetische Beratung.* Münster: Westfälisches Dampfboot.

Stock, G. (2000) Der Geist aus der Flasche: Soll die Gesellschaft die Entwicklung zur Genmanipulation stoppen – oder haben die Kinder von morgen nicht sogar ein Recht auf verbesserte Gene? *Spiegel*, 15: 190-192.

Weber, M. ([1920] 2000) *Die protestantische Ethik und der 'Geist' des Kapitalismus.* Weinheim: Beltz.

Weingart, P. (1989) 'Großtechnische Systeme': Ein Paradigma der Verknüpfung von Technologieentwicklung und Sozialem Wandel? in P. Weingart (Hg.) *Technik als sozialer Prozess.* Frankfurt am Main: Suhrkamp.

Wilmut, I. (2002) Klonen für medizinische Zwecke, *Spektrum der Wissenschaften: Dossier Gene, Klone, Fortpflanzung,* 4.

Appendix

Table: Facts and figures on assisted reproduction in Russia, Switzerland and Germany

Regulatory Situation			
Assisted reproductive technologies chiefly regulated by:	**Russia**	**Switzerland**	**Germany**
	Legislation basis for the protection of national health (1993); Family Law (1995); Special decree of Ministry of Health (2003)	Medical self-regulation (1981, 1985, 1990); Constitution (1993); Law [Fortpflanzungsmedizingesetz FMedG (2001), 'Law on reproductive medicine']	Law [Embryonenschutzgesetz ESG (1990), 'Law on the protection of embryos']; Medical self regulation (Bundesärztekammer BÄK, current version 2006)
Surrogacy	Legal Restricted to married couples	Illegal	Illegal (ESG)
Egg donation	Legal	Illegal	Illegal (ESG)
Sperm donation	Legal Right to know donor's identity is not debated	Legal Restricted to married couples Right to know donor's identity at age 18, but no possibility of parenthood claims	Legal No donor anonymity (possibility of legal parenthood claims towards donor) Only available if homologue treatment has been tried, but failed, and only after counselling Extremely reluctantly applied to unmarried couples, and never with homosexual couples or singles (BÄK). Never paid by health insurance
PGD	Legal but purely commercial	Illegal but currently being legalised (FMedG)	Illegal (ESG)

Regulatory Situation (cont.)			
Cloning	**Russia**	**Switzerland**	**Germany**
	Illegal, five year moratorium (2002). Today's official status is ambiguous	Illegal (constitution)	Illegal (ESG)
Preservation	Embryos: legal but with some restrictions Egg cells, sperm, pro-nuclei: legal	Embryos: illegal Egg cells, sperm, pro-nuclei (5 years): legal	Embryos: illegal except in exceptional circumstances (BÄK) Egg cells, sperm, pro-nuclei: legal (BÄK)
Time limits	Issue is not problematised	Embryos must be transferred as soon as medically possible.	Embryos must be transferred as soon as medically possible.
Age limits	Issue is not problematised	Patients must not be too old to be able to provide for child.	In relation to public health insurance payments: women 25-40, men 25-50
Other access restrictions	Issue is not problematised	Heterosexual couples only	Access restricted to heterosexual couples 'indirectly' by restricting access to sperm donation (above) and by making egg donation and surrogacy illegal
Indication	Only to treat infertility, or AI if a sexual partner is absent	Only to treat infertility, or to prevent transmission of serious heritable disease	Only to treat infertility, or to prevent transmission of serious heritable disease

Regulatory Situation (cont.)

Financing	**Russia**	**Switzerland**	**Germany**
	State pays for one cycle of insemination, but the amount of quotas is restricted and depends on the region.	Health insurance pays for diagnosis and up to three cycles of insemination, but not for IVF.	Since 2004, health insurance pays 50% of treatment costs for up to three cycles of IVF, but only if: - the patients are married - no donor sperm is involved - the patients are between 25 and 40 (women) and 50 (men) years of age - the couple submitted to counselling
hES research	Legal	Legal (2004)	Research is legal on imported stem cells. Generation of hES in Germany is illegal (Law for ensuring the protection of embryos in relation with hES imports and research, 2002).
Firsts	IVF: First birth in Moscow in February 1986; in St. Petersburg in September 1986	First IVF pregnancy in Basle, 1982; first birth in Locarno, 1984	1982: Oliver, in Erlangen

Numbers			
Treatment numbers (IVF, ICSI, fresh and cryo-cycles)	**Russia**	**Switzerland**	**Germany**
	2003: 11,000 IVF procedures	2007: 5,481 patients, 8,797 IVF/ICSI cycles	2007: 42,306 patients, 64,578 IVF/ICSI cycles
Percentages	Statistics unavailable	2006: 1.65% of all live births were conceived by ARTs (1,415 babies in total)	2006: 1.60% of all live births were conceived by ARTs (10,775 babies in total)
Success rates	2006: approximately 30-35% of IVF treatment cycles achieved pregnancies	2007: 23% of IVF/ICSI treatment cycles (including cryo-cycles) achieved pregnancies	2007: 22.1% of IVF/ICSI treatment cycles (including cryo-cycles) achieved pregnancies
Number of clinics	2005: 50	2007: 25	2007: 118

Sources: see chapters under 'National regimes of reproductive technologies'

About the authors

Bettina Bock von Wülfingen is an Assistant Professor at the Institute for Cultural Studies, Humboldt-Universität zu Berlin. During her doctoral research on health and illness in discourses on new reproductive and genetic technologies, she received different international visiting fellowships within Science and Technology Studies, working inter alia at IAS-STS in Graz/Austria; SATSU in York; and the BIOS centre in London. Her second book project deals with the history and methodology of the life sciences.

Olga Brednikova is a research fellow at the Centre for Independent Social Research in St. Petersburg, Russia, and head of the centre's research focus 'Borders and frontier communities'. She is the author of about fifty publications. Her current research interests include assisted reproductive technologies; nation-state borders and borderland spaces; migration; the sociology of everyday life; and qualitative methodology in sociology.

Willemijn de Jong is an Associate Professor of Social Anthropology at the University of Zurich. She teaches in the fields of kinship, family, gender, the body and technology, social security and contemporary social theory. She has published on migration and communication in Switzerland; textile work; marriage and gender; ritual revival and transformation in Flores, Indonesia; social security and ageing in Kerala, India; and recently on reproductive technologies and kinship in Euro-American contexts.

Andrea Früh holds an MA in Pedagogy and Social Anthropology from the University of Zurich. Her MA thesis focuses on individual coping strategies of Swiss women who used in vitro fertilisation and other reproductive technologies to become a parent. She was employed in a research and consultancy company in London. Currently she is working as a counselor in a refuge for women in Switzerland and as a journalist.

Nadya Nartova is a research associate at the Centre for Independent Social Research and a PhD candidate at the European University in St. Petersburg, Russia. Her research interests are in the fields of sociology of the body and sexuality; reproductive technologies; gender studies and feminist theory. She has authored numerous publications and is co-editor of two collections of articles on the body, sexuality and new technologies.

Zora Schaad graduated in Social Anthropology and Social and Preventive Medicine at the University of Zurich. Her MA thesis, entitled 'Finally parents: Influences of Reproductive Technologies and the Experience of Involuntary Childlessness on the Transition to Parenthood', dealt with the influences of reproductive medicine on social practices and cultural ideas of prospective parents. She is currently working as a journalist.

Shahanah Schmid studied Sociology, Social Anthropology and Pedagogy at the University of Zurich. Currently she is a PhD student in the BIOS centre, at the London School of Economics. Her PhD research is entitled 'Reproductive Medicine in Context: Knowledge Cultures of IVF in German Speaking Switzerland'. It focuses on local specificities of IVF discourses and how they relate to local imagery of the nation, gender and kinship.

Olga Tkach holds a PhD in Sociology. Her thesis deals with multi-generational families in the Russian factory milieu. She is currently working as a research fellow at the Centre for Independent Social Research in St. Petersburg, Russia. She has published about twenty articles related to historical sociology; gender studies; migration; and the sociology of everyday life. She has received several international visiting fellowships, and worked at the LSE in London; the Heinrich-Böll-Stiftung in Berlin; and the Fafo in Oslo.